THE NATURAL

How To Maximise Your Performance By Adopting a Natural Lifestyle

FOREWORD
By
JAN de VRIES
(World-Renowned Naturopath)

Master The Art of Running by Malcolm Balk

theartofrunning.com

www.evolution.running.com

David Reavely Cert Ed., Bed(Hons), FA(Cert)

ACKNOWLEDGEMENTS

I would like to thank everyone who has helped me in one way or another to bring this book to fruition, including my mother Iris, and my father Albert, (now both sadly deceased); my sister, Iris and her husband Jacky for their relentless encouragement; my wife, Lorraine, for her support and for having initiated me into the world of word processing. Also Jackie McGahey as she inspired me to persevere in my attempts to complete this book, and without her infectious encouragement, enthusiasm and computer skills it would merely be an unfulfilled idea. Many thanks also to Sasa Jankovic, magazine editor and freelance journalist, for her professional guidance and to Penguin UK and the magazine Health Guardian for their permission to publish extracts which appear in this book.

It should also be acknowledged that permission was sought for the extract from the book, 'Keep Healthy Stay Younger' by H Baker.

I would also like to mention my daughter Josie, who created the delightful illustrations.

Finally, I owe so much to Jan de Vries, for his kindness, guidance and expertise.

FOREWORD

I feel very honoured and complimented to write a foreword for this book. Dave and I have known each other for many years; I have always admired the way that he was interested in health during the period when he was teaching at a school for children with special needs. I was also encouraged by the way he helped young people by giving them the knowledge of a good healthy diet.

Dave has also been interested in sports and there is not a lot of material written for sports people, he has looked into this and with a lot of knowledge, advised those involved in sport to get the best out of good health.

This book is a book for the future and for those who shall live for the future in better health. It gives a lot of simple but very useful advice and in terms of achieving optimal function of one's capability, it shows how much can be achieved when one adheres to good dietary management.

I have been encouraged by reading this book for the simple reason that over the years, whilst working in this field, I too have seen that with good dietary management and good healthy living, how much the body will give – in other words, we get out what we put in.

I have always been happy to share with Dave the tremendous world of sensible living and how much nature is capable of healing and we are both agreed that with some natural methods, one's health can be improved. This is achieved by creating the right conditions for the body and supplying it with the correct nourishment; hence we are able to activate the body's own generation system. In this way it is possible to overcome and if necessary cure ailments. Prevention is always better than cure in the approach to health.

I am pleased that Dave, with all his years of research, has shared his knowledge in this book, which can easily be understood and practically applied. I am convinced that this work will show many people some very healthy ways. It is an excellent way to improve one's health and get the best out of it. I am sure that this book will be a great success and will find a valuable place in many homes.

Jan de Vries D.Ho.med.,D.O.,M.R.O.,N.D.M.R.N.,D.Ac.M.B.Ac.A.

Front cover design by Nigel Bowley - Seelan Associates
Illustrations by Josephine Reavely

Other titles available from Diviniti Publishing Ltd., include
A Best selling Hypnosis cassette and CD. series by Glenn Harrold
A range of Self Help Guides to Emotional Freedom by Liz Adamson

This publication is designed to provide health educational data in regard to
the subject matter covered. It is a reference and experential work of general
interest and benefit to readers and is not intended to treat, diagnose or prescribe.
The information contained herein is in no way to be considered a substitute
for consultation with a competent health care professional. Skilled medical
opinion is advised on specific health complaints before any course of action is
taken.

CONTENTS

INTRODUCTION

For some time now I have felt that there was a need for me to write a book on nutrition for athletes. My primary aim is to pass on to others the lessons I have learned through sometimes hard and bitter experience, and it is this objective that supplied the inner motivation so necessary in tackling such a task.

It could be said that an increasing number of people in this country are becoming aware of the vital need for more natural foods, and with it the desire for a better and well balanced diet. This is evidenced by the tremendous growth of the health food industry, which is after all, purely indicative of the demand for foods nearer to their natural state, since without consumer demand no industry could thrive and grow. In my own opinion, I feel that this is also an indication that the public are becoming more aware of the dangers of our so called 'modern civilised diet' so predominant in this and other countries. However, I feel that it is also true to say that much ignorance concerning correct nutrition still abounds, and it has been my experience that this applies no less to our present day sportsmen and women, who although sometimes familiar with complex scientific training programmes, body mechanics (or kinetics) and progressive weight training schedules for specific needs, are almost totally ignorant of their bodies' requirements in relation to correct nutrition as constituted by a properly balanced diet. The human body when healthy is like a well tuned engine - all it requires to keep it 'ticking over' is healthy exercise, plenty of rest, fresh air, water, the right mental approach and the correct fuel; or in other words with regard to the latter, an abundance of natural foods designed by nature to fulfil the body's demands for protein, carbohydrate, roughage, fats and a combination of vitamins and minerals, all in their correct balance.

Providing that the foregoing factors are all present, the body will run at an optimum level of efficiency, as indeed it was designed to do under such circumstances. For the sportsman and sportswoman, as we shall discover later in this chapter, these facts are of vital importance.

As a teacher of physical education and football coach, I have had ample opportunity to assess present day attitudes towards conditioning and general physical training for those engaged in sport at various levels. My regretful opinion is that although much has been achieved in terms of improving performance, largely through the applied techniques of scientifically based weight training schedules and superior training facilities, etc, conversely, the science of nutrition, as applied to the physical needs of the individual, has been largely neglected.

In a sense then, this book is my answer to a very definite need - that of providing information on how to eat for health and the achievement of better physical performance in whatever the chosen sport.

In addition, it is my belief that if a natural mode of living is adopted by sports people, then not only will their chances of achieving an optimum level of performance be enhanced, but their capacity to perform over a longer period in terms of fitness and stamina will also be greatly increased. When we observe the physical condition of people who live in a natural environment, existing on a diet consisting of mainly fruits, vegetables and other natural foods, then we may conclude that such a premise is not without scientific foundation.

Undoubtedly, there is still much confusion in the minds of the public concerning the merits of specific diets and foods, the controversy over cholesterol and the possible dangers associated with genetically modified foods. That such confusion and controversy exists is to be expected, since the subject of nutrition is an extremely complex one. I have, therefore, attempted to present the reader with certain dietary principles, because regardless of the complexities of the subject, it is obvious that there are certain laws which apply to the human race as a species. Moreover, it stands to reason that by adhering to a lifestyle which is based upon these natural laws, then sporting prowess may be enhanced and indeed prolonged.

8

Research by a number of eminent scientists such as Sir Robert McCarrison and Dr. Bircher Benner would seem to indicate that our modern sophisticated diet is responsible for a great deal of the ill health so prevalent in the world today. But what does our present-day diet consist of that is seemingly so detrimental to health and in what way is this significant to those who are engaged in sport on a serious or not so serious level? The answer to these and other questions will be dealt with in the forthcoming chapters of this book.

In order to relate to you the importance of a natural diet in my own case, and how I arrived at the decision to write this book, it is important that I provide you with a brief account of the events which changed my life quite drastically for the better.

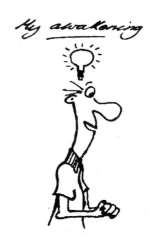

CHAPTER 1   MY AWAKENING

I remember that particular period in my childhood very clearly. I was about thirteen years of age, and like any other normal child, simply bursting with energy. I found my physical outlets in soccer, swimming, running, cycling and anything that provided me with pure and undiluted activity! I seemed to thrive on movement and seldom felt tired despite the rigours that my body was almost incessantly subjected to.

I don't know when the first symptoms began to manifest themselves, but I suspect that at first it was easier for me to shrug them off and pretend that nothing was wrong. My left knee began to swell and show a little discomfort, usually after a hard game of football or after a long walk. At the time I thought little of it, but for a child of thirteen 'bathed' in blissful ignorance of such maladies as arthritis, that was to be expected. It was merely discomfort and an interference at the time.

My active lifestyle continued and the natural energy that I possessed refused to be stifled. At the time it appeared that nothing would stop me. However, the symptoms continued and progressively grew worse. In the past, after a strenuous game of football my left knee would swell and become a little stiff, the symptoms gradually disappearing with time. Now, however, the swelling was more pronounced, the stiffness harder to ignore and the pain quite acute.

It was soon apparent that something had to be done. A visit to my doctor was the first step and eventually a consultation with a local specialist.

The specialist did not take long to diagnose the problem, and I remember the word 'arthritis' being uttered, though I was never directly informed what this meant. My father, who had accompanied me to the hospital was told that 'your son is too active!', and that my leg was to be immobilised in plaster for 'several weeks'.

I look back at that day with some amusement; all that concerned me was the fact that my leg was to be put in plaster, and far from worrying about this state of affairs, in a perverse kind of way I was delighted about it! I suppose I thought of my newly acquired plaster as a sort of status symbol. Undoubtedly I would be the centre of attention amongst my friends at school for a while. I think that my father was quite taken aback by my lack of concern over the situation, but I could observe a distinct hint of amusement in his eyes as he observed my reaction.

That plaster may have immobilised my leg, but it certainly didn't immobilise me! My cycle of activity continued, although slowed down somewhat. I was a perfect example of human adaptation, as I quickly and eagerly adjusted to riding a bicycle using one leg and playing a sort of monoped football.

After what appeared to be an eternity, the time came to have the plaster removed. It was in fact with a mixture of curiosity and partial regret that I viewed the situation that day - curiosity as to what my leg would look like after several weeks of entombment and regret that I would be losing such a prominent status symbol. Afterwards the verdict was given; the swelling in my knee had subsided and mobility was normal, the treatment had been a success - or so it seemed. For several years I carried on with my active lifestyle, although slowing down a little as maturity approached. Eventually, by the time I was fifteen I had added another activity to my growing list of sporting pursuits - that of weightlifting. As with my other interests I threw myself into this new physical endeavour wholeheartedly. Training at the Sunderland Y.M.C.A. under the dedicated guidance of a qualified weightlifting coach, I was quick to acquire the necessary skills and soon reached the stage at which I could participate in weightlifting exhibitions. By the time I was seventeen, my name had appeared several times in local newspapers which served to further heighten my interest and enthusiasm for the sport.

It is difficult to assess at just what stage in my teens that the then long-forgotten symptoms of arthritis made themselves painfully obvious to me once again. If I remember correctly I was nineteen at the time and just beginning to enjoy the publicity that was coming my way as a result of my weightlifting endeavours.

In the past I was not unduly concerned with the implications of my discomfort, now however, I was older and wiser, and it didn't take me long to realise the seriousness of the situation. To a young man whose life revolved around activity, it was a bitter blow indeed!

My knee trouble, which again comprised of swelling and discomfort, would come and go. But it was becoming increasingly difficult to ignore. As time progressed so did the symptoms, until at times I was literally crippled with pain. Something had to be done, but what? Most people knew that arthritis was classed as an incurable disease in the eyes of the medical profession. Was I therefore doomed to a life of painful activity as an arthritic cripple? Certainly everything seemed to indicate this to be the case, since the symptoms were now beginning to make themselves manifest in my right knee also. I was depressed and fearful of the future; why couldn't I be like other boys of my age without cares and worries about health? Surely arthritis was something that affected people when they reached middle-age and older; was not my father a perfect example of this state of affairs. A joiner by profession he had been afflicted with arthritis in the worst possible part of his body from his point of view - his hands! Perhaps then my health problems had been inherited, and if so it seemed that my chances of recovery would be even slimmer.

As a teenager one of my favourite subjects at school was biology. Somehow I found this subject fascinating and it wasn't long before I excelled at it. Perhaps it was my natural curiosity towards the human body and its functions that encouraged me to seek for an answer through nutrition, or it may have been an element of pure chance that led my enquiring mind in that direction. Whatever the reason behind my new interest, I was soon eagerly pursuing the idea of health foods as the antidote to my illness. Here then was an approach towards my problem which offered me something that the orthodox medical profession could not - hope!

As with my various sporting activities I threw myself into the subject of nutrition with the genuine enthusiasm of a person who has just been given real hope for the future. I soon found myself eating less white bread and white sugar, tinned and packaged foods dosed with preservatives, emulsifiers and colourants became a thing of the past. Instead, I made weekly pilgrimages to the local health food shop in order to buy wholewheat bread, molasses, honey, muesli, brown rice and flour milled from organically-grown wheat. It was all a new and fascinating world to me, and I was eager to try everything!

After persevering for some weeks however, the arthritis was still evident and I caught just as many colds and other infections as everyone else, despite my much improved eating habits. Why? I asked myself, surely I must be doing something fundamentally wrong?

Further research seemed to be the logical answer. Subsequently my

13

desire was for further knowledge, since I really believed that a nutritional approach had to offer a solution to my problem.

Soon my incessant demand for further knowledge was to bring results. There was, I discovered, a completely different system of medicine being used to treat arthritis and similar chronic diseases, not only in Britain but throughout the world. This system, known as **naturopathy** used a nutritional approach towards disease. Its philosophy encompassed delving into the individual lifestyle of the patient and attempting to get to the root cause of the trouble. I read numerous books on the subject and learned much in a short space of time.

Armed with a new knowledge on the subject of nutrition as an approach towards curing disease, I was again ready to effect a change of lifestyle with renewed vigour. This time, instead of making the mistake of consuming natural foods indiscriminately, I began to balance my diet so that it was predominately alkaline-forming; as this was in accordance with naturopathic principles. The result, although not immediate, was nevertheless quite incredible! All signs of arthritic symptoms began to disappear. I felt fitter, looked healthier, and whilst other people suffered frequently from colds and 'flu, I remained seemingly impervious. My new way of life had been changed dramatically for the better. Not without sacrifice or without an element of mental turmoil in the beginning when things didn't work out. Nevertheless, with all of this behind me, I was now free in mind and body; and it was so wonderful to be able to swim, train with heavy weights and participate in numerous other physical activities without fearing the consequences. And all of this through a change of lifestyle involving diet.

At this stage I would forgive the reader for asking a very pertinent question: "What has all of this got to do with nutrition and physical performance?" My answer is simple; the dietary approach which I used to overcome arthritis and subsequently restore maximum bodily efficiency, both in terms of fitness and health (remembering that the two are not necessarily synonymous, since a fit person can be unhealthy), is equally relevant to the sportsman and sportswoman. In essence, this is because a lifestyle which will help to promote good health (and thus freedom from disease), and maximise efficiency of the body and all its constituent parts, must in turn help to promote improved physical performance in whatever the chosen sport. The motto is clear, the human body cannot perform at its best if it is hampered by anything less than optimum physiological efficiency. Such a degree of efficiency is seldom fully achieved by anyone, but the nearer one can get towards attaining such a goal, the better the physical performance of the person in question; in whatever the chosen sport.

Furthermore, and equally important, it has been my sad experience that the majority of sports participants today are almost totally ignorant when it comes to following sensible eating habits. I firmly believe that the situation exists in which considerable harm is being done to people's health. On the surface this may seem ridiculous to the average person unacquainted with sensible eating practices. However, I would suggest that the effects of long-term indiscriminate eating habits are far from obvious, the damage being brought about over a period of years. For example, there are a number of high-class athletes and footballers around today who are constantly suffering from one injury after another and no doubt questioning why, after years of optimum efficiency, their highly-tuned bodies are beginning to let them down. Usually the common explanation is 'Oh he or she must be past their peak'. In this respect I don't disagree that ageing will inevitably take its toll on human performance. However, as a number of practitioners of alternative medicine will confirm, an increasing number of top-class sportsmen and sportswomen are seeking advice about repeated injuries and illness, only to discover that it is their lifestyle that is at fault and not so much the physical demands placed upon their bodies.

This point was brought home to me recently when engaged in a conversation with a physical training instructor in the south of England. It transpired that he had just returned from a course on physical fitness and one component of the course had been the importance of adhering to a natural diet in order to improve and maintain maximum physical performance. Conversely, it was suggested that a number of top athletes in this country were ending their careers prematurely as a result of adhering to a 'junk' food diet. This was most interesting to me because it served to illustrate that some of this country's fitness experts were beginning to take notice of this possibility.

This book, therefore, does not merely concern itself with enhancing physical performance, but also in improving dietary habits designed to further the health of the individual, and thus lay down a path that leads towards a healthier lifestyle.

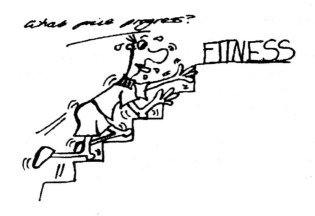

CHAPTER 2   WHAT PRICE PROGRESS?

Man, from the very beginning of his evolution has had to rely upon the natural environment for his supply of food. Primarily a hunter and gatherer, he depended mainly on wild game for his protein and fat, wild herbs and fruit for his vitamins, minerals and medicines, and honey for his energy-supplying sugars. As he evolved further, so he became less inclined to devote almost his entire energy towards hunting; instead he channelled his energies in the direction of farming. His constantly improving skills in farming resulted in better food yields. So much so in fact, that he had to store such items as cereals, meat and vegetables. The effect of this transition was dramatic! For the first time homo sapiens had time on his hands. No longer did he have to spend his days hunting, gathering and merely surviving in a hostile environment. Now there was a food surplus, not so much that he could afford to sit back and relax of course, but just enough to give him more time; and with time, the opportunity to think; and thus the opportunity to invent. Gradually mankind became more complex; small settlements grew into towns and the towns into cities. After farming methods developed even more (especially after the invention of the wheel), once again food yields increased, and with the surplus of food came a surplus in population, which in turn resulted in bigger communities. This spiralling process has continued until the present day, with our huge towns and cities, and vast networks of roadways and railways, etc.

Even now, in a world as technically and scientifically advanced as ours, there remain living reminders of our primitive past. In Australia, for example, the Aborigine has quickly become 'infected' with the 'germ' of technical progress. But there are still tribes around the world who live as we once did, living the life-cycle of the hunter/gatherer. Left to their own devices, these people may well evolve as we did, although much depends upon what environmental resources are available.

One of the important facts to emerge from any study of the historical background of mankind, is the reality that up until the last few hundred years, people have lived very close to nature when it came to consumption of food. The majority of foodstuffs were untampered with. Flour, for instance was of the wholemeal variety, and contained its full complement of vitamins, proteins, minerals, enzymes, carbohydrates and fibre; the common sweetener was either molasses (the crude product of the sugar cane, rich in minerals and natural sugars), honey or dried fruit. Cheese was free from emulsifiers and remained unprocessed, and milk was raw and unpasteurised. The interesting situation presently exists in which these foods of the past; which were taken so much for granted and consumed daily, are now regarded as so-called health foods, and remain the exception rather than the norm.

Instead of living on these untampered foods, designed by nature to fulfil the body's requirements for sustenance, repair and resistance to disease, our present day society now lives on such 'foodless' foods as white flour (a substance consisting mostly of starch and chemical additives, the nutritious wheatgerm and fibre having been removed), white sugar, a multitude of convenience, tinned and packaged foods with their vast array of dyes, preservatives, emulsifiers, improvers and numerous other questionable chemical additives, in addition to a whole host of other refined and adulterated substances designed for human consumption, and which can only loosely be described as food.

18

Mankind has indeed progressed in certain respects, but it is nevertheless something of a paradox that our progression has led to regression! In terms of feeding habits this is no less true.

Modern day scientific research has uncovered convincing evidence that the complex diet of civilised countries is a major causative factor in producing such insidious chronic complaints as heart disease, certain cancers, diabetes and numerous other human afflictions.

This has now received official recognition from government experts in several countries around the world. For example, in the early 1980s two government reports were produced in this country; namely the COMA AND NACNE Reports, both of which highlighted the deficiencies within the average British diet. In addition to this it also made a number of recommendations concerning dietary improvements. In essence, these reports recommended the following:

1. A reduction of sugar and salt.
2. An increase in consumption of high fibre, unprocessed foods, such as wholegrains, fruits and vegetables.
3. A reduction of fat intake, particularly saturated fats.

Interestingly enough, a report by W.H.O (The World Health Organisation) published in 1991; strongly recommends a dramatic increase in people's consumption of fresh fruit and vegetables.

The point here of course, is that these reports further substantiate what nature-cure practitioners have been advocating for many years, namely that in order to reduce the number of diseases that afflict us, we must revert to a more natural diet. The fact that the situation is now receiving official recognition from governments from around the world is perhaps an encouraging step in the right direction.

If you are truly concerned with keeping your body at the peak of efficiency, or merely hope to attain or maintain a certain level of health and fitness throughout life, then the advice laid down in the ensuing chapters of this book may be of tantamount importance.

In this regard, *George H. Baker* in his excellent book *'Keep Healthy Stay Younger'*, has this to say concerning the diet of present-day athletes:

> 'Even the exceptional muscular strength possessed by some men is not a safeguard against sickness and disease. Examples of this are quite readily found amongst the apparently superbly fit athletes, footballers, weightlifters, boxers, wrestlers, swimmers and others. The relatively high rate of colds and influenza would suggest that in spite of the excellent physical fitness of these men, something must be wrong for them to get illnesses such as these common ailments. Exposure to the cold and wet with footballers cannot be the basic cause, for indoor athletes get colds and 'flu and other common disorders. The basic cause would logically appear to be in the food they eat.'
>
> Baker, H, 1975, Keep Healthy Stay Younger, Sphere Books.

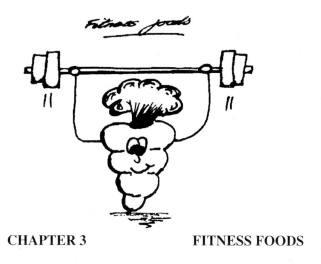

CHAPTER 3   **FITNESS FOODS**

On numerous occasions in the past I have had sportsmen and sportswomen ask me the question "What does a natural diet consist of?" My answer is usually the same - it very much depends upon the specific needs of the individual, since each person's food requirements will vary according to the chosen sport or sports. Obviously the weightlifter who is engaged in lifting heavy weights and is thus working his overall musculature in a severe manner, will have different protein requirements compared to a volleyball player for instance. Nonetheless, there is one basic principle that one should observe when undergoing the transition from a 'junk' food diet to a more natural one. In essence, an element of common sense is required when selecting food. For instance, when offered a choice between a tin of pears heavily sweetened with white sugar syrup and a pound of fresh pears, one would choose the latter; since the tinned product has been adulterated with sugar and possibly contaminated with other dubious additives as well; neither of which are likely to be beneficial to the body. Similarly, if there is a choice between white bread, which consists predominately of starch and contains a number of chemical additives, and the wholewheat variety, which contains the nutritious wheatgerm, fibre and is free of additives; once again, one would select the latter.

This element of distinction between natural and unnatural foods must be at the forefront of the judicious buyer's mind. The path is not an easy one, especially when the majority of people around you are feeding on the commonly accepted foods of society. Certainly in such a situation you will be open to criticism. However, the majority of criticism aimed at you will be born out of ignorance. People seldom like to be confronted with the concept that their diet, which has been accepted as a matter of course sometimes over many years, is fundamentally in question.

Many times I have been assailed with the question "Why don't you eat normal food like the rest of us?" I usually agree that it is indeed normal food, but only normal in the sense that the majority of people eat it. It is with this thought in mind that I would like to remind the reader of the foregoing statement from chapter 2 "These foods of the past, which were taken so much for granted and consumed daily, are now regarded as so-called 'health foods', and remain the exception rather than the norm."

For a growing number of people, therefore, it would appear that a complete circle of public attitude is in evidence. This is perhaps progressing at a very slow rate, but is nevertheless significant, as illustrated by the following diagram:

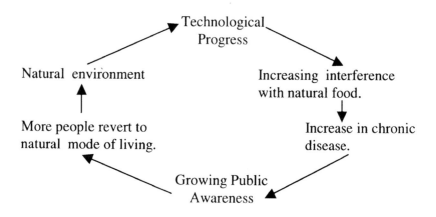

Growing public awareness.

The proof that we have come full circle in terms of how we perceive natural foods is very much reflected by consumer demand. This is very obvious when we consider the increased availability of organic foods. After all, who would have believed just a few years ago that customers could walk around almost any major supermarket in the country and literally fill a shopping trolley with an array of organic fruit, vegetables, pre-packaged foods, fruit juices, honey, cheese, cereals and so forth.

When I first began purchasing so called health foods in the 1970s, organic produce was rare. I even had to visit my local allotments in Sunderland in order to seek out gardeners who grew produce without chemicals, or at least kept their use to a minimum. The fruit and vegetables that I brought home with me were magnificent, not only in terms of appearance, but also because of their wonderful flavour - a common characteristic of naturally grown fruits and vegetables.

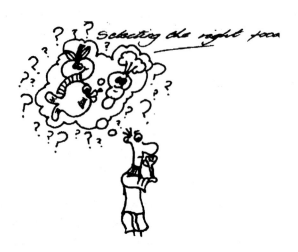

SELECTING THE RIGHT FOODS

Shown below is a table of foods designed to illustrate to the reader the kind of choice that is required if a natural diet is to be followed with conviction:

OMIT THESE	OPT FOR
White flour and everything. made from it	Wholewheat flour and products made from it such as biscuits and wholemeal bread.
White rice, spaghetti, etc.	Choose instead wholemeal spaghetti, pasta and rice.
White sugar and its products.	Honey, molasses, black treacle and dark brown sugar in moderation.

Dried fruit, preserved with mineral oils, sulphur dioxide, etc.	Unpreserved dried fruit - available from health food stores.
Refined breakfast cereals.	Muesli, porridge, wholewheat cereals.
Processed cheese.	Unprocessed cheese free from artificial additives. Cottage cheese is a good alternative.
Artificially flavoured drinks.	Unsweetened fruit and vegetable juices such as apple, orange and grape (preferably organically grown).
Fried and greasy foods, such as burgers and chips	Foods dressed in natural vegetable oils such as sunflower or lightly cooked in olive oil.
Sweetened tinned fruit.	Soaked dried fruit (rich in natural energy-giving sugars), such as dates, figs, raisins and sultanas. These should be organically grown where possible.
Coffee and tea.	Herb teas, sweetened with honey if preferred; dandelion coffee or similar substitute.
Heavily spiced foods such as sauces pickles, malt vinegar, etc.	Natural herbs (example bay, sage and mint), mild spices in moderation. Cider vinegar is a good substitute for ordinary vinegar.

Rich and fatty meats, tinned meats.	Chicken and organ meats such as heart, liver and kidney. Preferably from naturally reared animals.
Meals rich in carbohydrate and little else.	Meals balanced between starchy foods (eg. potatoes) with freshly cooked vegetables and protein rich foods.

The foregoing list could be extended almost indefinitely, but since it is my purpose to deal with the fundamental principles behind choosing a correct diet, as well as attempting to make clear the path that leads towards a generally improved lifestyle designed to enhance health and fitness, I will end this table here with the hope that I have at least stimulated the reader into thinking about his/her eating habits and how they could be improved.

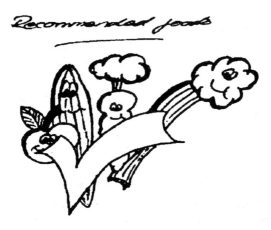

RECOMMENDED FOODS

It is my intention here to deal with certain specifically recommended foods, renowned for their value in helping to promote health and currently being used by numerous sports people as an aid towards the achievement of greater levels of fitness.

Obviously these foods will not improve fitness on their own. However, in my opinion they can provide a vital 'cog in the living machine of efficiency'. The serious athlete or the sports participant merely concerned with maintaining a certain degree of well-being and fitness, can be helped towards this end, if close attention is paid towards careful dietary planning. Few athletes, irrespective of their ability, can thrive for long on poor nutrition; eventually the signs of failing performance will show through. A number of modern day examples of this state of affairs are in evidence today.

There will always be the exception to the rule, however, and a classic example is the athlete who 'burns the candle at both ends' - living it up to the small hours, drinking heavily the night before an important competition or game, and eating everything in sight regardless of the consequences. When it comes to a test of his athletic ability and endurance, he still manages to do well. To the person who adheres to a sensible life-style it can be sickening! Usually the individual who can get away with the high living routine has an above-average constitution and their body will throw off poisons that would severely hamper most of us. Perhaps Rasputin was such a person, since apart from his above-average strength, it appears that his system could withstand a normally lethal dose of poison - much to the astonishment of his would-be killers! Nevertheless, even the exceptional constitution in question will often break-down in time after years of constant abuse; and who knows to what heights of greatness such a person might attain if he or she did follow a more natural mode of living and training.

For the majority, therefore, it is wise not to challenge nature's laws with impunity. Instead, we must learn to live in harmony with nature, and to help the reader to achieve this objective, I will now proceed to deal with the foods that have a reputation for enhancing health and fitness.

HONEY
Honey has been a valuable source of food to man for literally thousands of years. The earliest record of man's interest in this wonderful product of the bees dates back to Palaeolithic times. For instance, in a series of prehistoric rock paintings discovered at a place called Cuevas de la Arana in Spain, there is a scene in which men are shown plundering a wild bees nest. Man has always had an extremely high regard for this so-called 'Food of the Gods'. Indeed, several books have been written which deal entirely with the subject of honey, its history and properties.

From a nutritional point of view (and this is particularly relevant to the sports participant), honey is valued for its use as a rapid energy booster. Honey functions very much like ordinary sugar (sucrose) in that it raises what is known as the blood-sugar level, thus providing energy which is readily available to the body. Nevertheless, honey, unlike refined sugar is a complex substance containing vitamins, minerals, enzymes and wax. Moreover, honey contains a mixture of what are termed simple sugars, which are easily broken down by the digestive

28

system - the end result being an extremely quick and easily assimilated source of energy!

Despite the fact that the vitamins and minerals in honey are usually found in minute quantities, they are nonetheless still worthy of special note, knowing as we do that these trace elements in food are essential for normal body functioning even in tiny amounts.

Numerous experiments on honey both for its medicinal value and its importance as a source of food for sportsmen and women have been conducted throughout the world. As a source of almost instant energy, honey is highly esteemed, and subsequently is used by many athletes prior to competition, game or whenever a high demand for energy is required.

In conclusion, therefore, I am of the opinion that honey is worthy of mention as a health-giving and fitness-promoting food, and as such I feel that the reader would do well to make use of some of the suggestions for its use at the end of this section. Since the use of pesticides and other artificial chemicals on the land is so widespread, it may be advisable to select honey that has been harvested from pollution-free areas wherever feasible, for example, honey from African forests.

WHEATGERM

One of the most commonly consumed foods today is white flour in its variety of forms (eg. bread, biscuits, cakes, etc.). Few people are aware that this flour is a poor substitute for the wholewheat variety. In fact, although the situation is slowly changing, the majority of people still prefer to buy white bread instead of wholewheat simply because they have been 'brainwashed' into thinking that white bread is good for you and that the difference between the two is minimal.

I wonder just how many of these people would uphold this view if they knew a little of our modern milling process? Here is a brief description of what happens:

Firstly, the wheat grains are separated into three parts by mechanical steel rollers. Bran (useful as a source of fibre and some minerals and B vitamins), wheatgerm (rich in vitamins, enzymes, protein, etc.), and the white starchy endosperm. It is mainly the latter starch predominant endosperm that is used to make our popular white loaf. The majority of the wheatgerm and bran is fed to farm animals because they are known to thrive on these foods. However, the process is not finished yet, there are several chemical additives incorporated into the manufacture of white bread before it is deemed ready for human consumption!

The particular constituent of wheat that we are concerned with here is the wheatgerm. As the name suggests, this substance is known as the germ of the wheat, and it is very high in nutrients. Furthermore, since it contains the vital genetic information so necessary in furthering the species, it may well contain certain factors that have yet to be discovered. Of the most important constituents of wheatgerm, those worthy of note are protein, B vitamins, vitamin E and iron. All of these are important as factors which can influence health and fitness. Vitamin E for instance, is of particular interest at present and scientists continue to investigate its beneficial effects on the human body, especially as an aid towards strengthening the heart and circulatory system. It is also valuable as an antioxidant, helping to protect us from free radicals, which are unstable molecules produced by pollution, junk food, stress etc. They are circulated around the body causing damage to healthy cells.

Wheatgerm is regarded as one of the vitality foods and consequently may be worthy of note as an aid towards promoting sports performance. As a food, it can easily be incorporated into the everyday diet.

What to buy
There are a number of brands of wheatgerm on the market and to the health-minded buyer, the inevitable question will arise Which do I choose? . To simplify this matter wheatgerm can be divided into two categories, stabilised and unstabilised. Of the two, the former is lowest

in nutritional value, having been slightly toasted and vacuum packed in order to prevent its deterioration. The unstabilised variety is obviously better from a nutritional point of view, however, its great disadvantage is that it goes off very quickly indeed. What happens is that this type of wheatgerm reacts with the air and oxidises, or in simple terms turns rancid. Even unstabilised wheatgerm kept in a refrigerator in a sealed container will keep only a few days.

In actual fact, this tendency to deteriorate quickly is often a sign that the food in question has a high nutritional value. Usually we discover that the foods commonly termed vital or live foods, because of their natural vitality are the ones that are broken down by microbes and other environmental factors in the shortest space of time. These foods attract microbes like a magnet attracts iron, simply because they are rich in organic substances and are thus more attractive to micro-organisms of various kinds.

The choice of wheatgerm is ultimately up to the reader, but I would suggest that since the overall value of the stabilised variety is far from lost, then this would be the better choice.

WHEATGERM OIL

As the name suggests, this is oil which is derived from the wheatgerm itself. It is extremely valued by some athletes for its usefulness as a vitality booster. Experiments with animals for instance have indicated that physical stamina and overall cardiovascular fitness are influenced significantly when wheatgerm oil is included in the diet. Certainly it is extremely popular with a large number of athletes, particularly those involved in sports, where great stress is placed upon the cardiovascular system.

When buying wheatgerm oil one has a choice of capsules or the bottled oil. There seems little to choose between the two, but it is best to opt for the oil that has been cold pressed. This term indicates that oil has been derived without subjecting the wheatgerm to heat when in the process of extraction. Since the vitamins in wheatgerm, in particular vitamin E (for which wheatgerm is mostly prized) are easily subject to deterioration, the cold-pressing method results in less deterioration of the oil itself.

When buying wheatgerm oil, select oils which are sealed in dark stained bottles, since the vitamin E has a tendency to react with light. Once purchased, the bottle or similar container, should be stored in the refrigerator and used when required.

MOLASSES

As with the refining of wheat a similar story holds true with regard to the production of white sugar. At one end of the production line we have the sugar-cane; a plant rich in minerals, protein, vitamins, sucrose and fruit sugars. This sugar-cane is put through a variety of processes, from which white sugar is finally derived. The dark sticky syrup which is extracted from the sugar-cane at the beginning of the refining process is called molasses, which is, like wheatgerm and bran, fed livestock because they thrive on it. The next stage in the refining process produces black treacle, which like molasses is of good nutrient value, except it is higher in sucrose and consequently less bitter to taste. The next stage gives us golden syrup, which is of value as a sweetener only, having a very high sucrose content. Finally, white sugar is produced - a substance which is devoid of any real nutritional value and useful as a sweetener and energy provider only.

In terms of its mineral content, molasses is high in iron and another important mineral, potassium. It is also very useful as a supplier of B vitamins, which are involved in a whole range of bodily processes, such as digestion and nerve function. Perhaps because of its high potassium content it has been linked with cancer prevention. Sometimes molasses is given to domestic animals as a conditioner. Interestingly enough, my father once had a fascinating experience a number of years ago when using molasses. Being in his sixties at the time his hair had been grey for some time, as were his whiskers. I had persuaded him to take molasses because of its high nutrient content. After taking a tablespoonful every day for about a month, he was delighted to discover that his whiskers and sideburns had started to regain their original dark colour. Funnily enough however, the hair on his head remained grey.

In addition, evidence is presently accumulating which adds weight to the argument that white sugar is a major causative factor in bringing about the onset of diabetes and circulatory diseases. To the sports enthusiast, all of this is of vital importance of course, bearing in mind the aforementioned comments concerning the judicious selection of foods which are least interfered with by man.

Nature, in her wisdom has provided us with a substance that is extremely rich in essential nutrients in a readily assimilable form. It would be wrong of me to suggest that everyone should venture into their nearest health food store or chemist in order to buy molasses. It is not an essential food, nor is it even palatable to everyone, largely due to its bitter/sweet taste. Nevertheless, as a health and fitness-promoting food it is, I feel, worthy of mention.

FRUIT AND VEGETABLES

Most people, even those most ignorant of the value of a properly balanced diet, are aware that fruit and vegetables are good for you. In fact, to the health-conscious individual who is aware of naturopathic principles, fruit and vegetables are of supreme importance indeed.

A diet based largely on the daily consumption of fruit and vegetables (particularly when the majority of these foods are eaten in their raw state) will provide us with a good supply of vitamins, minerals, and various other important food factors. But this is not all, because these natural products of the earth are also valued for their cleansing and blood-building properties.

To the under-par or sick body, fruit and vegetables are good news. The food factors in such foods as apples, pears, carrots, cucumber, parsley, leeks, onions, garlic, swede and beetroot; are used by the body for its sustenance and repair; and in building a powerful resistance to disease.

In health the blood is slightly alkaline. However, if a person lives on a diet of indiscriminately selected foods, there is a tendency for the blood to become too acidic. This is primarily due to the consumption of too many acid-forming foods. A classic example of such a diet would be the typical high refined carbohydrate/protein diet so prevalent in our modern society. For instance a meal comprising of meat, chips, white bread with a stodgy pudding and a cup of tea to follow, is predominately acid-forming. This is because most of the foods in question produce acid waste-products during the process of digestion. Conversely, foods such as oranges, grapes, apples and pears, enter the system as acids but are converted to alkalis. Alkaline salts that are produced as a result of digestion are very important, since they not only help to nourish the system but also help to cleanse the body of unwanted toxins. The relevance to the reader, irrespective of whether he or she is interested in improving physical performance, or simply concerned with building or maintaining a feeling of well-being and fitness is clear. Physiological efficiency can only be achieved providing that the body is in a state of physical and mental homeostasis. In other words, so long as the body receives the basic requirements as mentioned in the foregoing pages, comprising of exercise, rest, correct mental balance and a properly constituted diet, then maximum efficiency in relation to fitness and health is far more likely to be achieved.

The role of fruit and vegetables in facilitating this is not insignificant, since a group of foods that have the reputation of helping to maintain and where necessary restore a body back to health, must surely figure prominently in the diet of all those who are engaged in sport. I do not base these conclusions on mere second-hand knowledge, but on my own experience. It was, in fact, through the act of changing my diet so that it was predominately alkaline-forming, that resulted in an amazing transformation in my body which ultimately brought about the complete cessation of arthritic symptoms. This in itself prevented the gradual physical deterioration that would have ensued had my whole lifestyle not been revolutionised.

In conclusion, therefore, fruit and vegetables represent a major cornerstone in the diet of all those engaged in sporting activities. In my own experience, I have discovered that whenever I consistently follow a diet of mostly fruit and vegetables (a large proportion of which are organically grown) then my stamina and general physical efficiency are at their peak. This is especially noticeable when I play vigorous sports such as five-a-side football, when at the age of 47 I am able to compete with men who are in their twenties and thirties. In fact, sometimes fellow players will comment on my ability to equal and often exceed the work rate of much younger footballers.

Interestingly enough, when the converse situation exists and I have been bingeing on junk food (yes, I'm human too!) then my performance is sluggish and my joints sore and prone to injury.

BREWER'S YEAST

This food is worthy of mention because it is not only rich in protein, but also the complete range of B vitamins, otherwise referred to as the B complex.

The B vitamins that make up the B complex have been carefully studied by scientists. It has been discovered that each B vitamin has a different function, however, it is important to remember that they all work together. Yeast is a minute cultivated plant about one four thousandth of an inch in diameter. It is comparable in size to a human blood corpuscle.

Brewer's yeast is grown under carefully controlled conditions in large vats until it has produced the greatest number of yeast cells. It is then collected and dried at a given temperature, which ensures that it retains its nutritional value.

Yeast is rich in many food factors, in fact, in addition to being rich in B vitamins, it contains sixteen of the twenty amino-acids which are the building blocks for tissue replacement in the body, and essential for normal body functioning. It also contains calcium, iron and ten trace minerals.

How To Take Yeast

Since yeast has a tendency to form gas in the digestive system, you would be well advised to take it in small quantities at first. Do not select live yeast in any form as this has a tendency to grow in the intestines and actually use up the body's supply of B vitamins. Brewer's yeast is perfectly safe, however, as it is no longer active. The exception to this rule would be the person who suffers from the condition known as candidiasis, which is a yeast infection that proliferates in the intestines bringing about all manner of symptoms from headaches to colitis. In such people it would be wise to omit yeast from the diet. If unsure, seek advice from a reputable natural health practitioner, such as a naturopath or nutritional consultant.

As yeast is a concentrated food, being very rich in protein (it contains twice as much protein pound for pound as meat), it can be a valuable addition to the diet of people engaged in sport. It is said that a heaped tablespoonful of yeast will supply twenty grammes of protein. One can conclude, therefore, that yeast is one of the cheapest forms of protein available.

What To Choose

Yeast comes in two forms - powder or tablets (aside from liquid yeast based preparations). The powder is useful in that it can be added to soups, baking, drinks, etc. However, not everyone likes the taste of yeast and to these people, swallowing tablets may be preferable. You can buy yeast from most chemists and health food stores. Remember though to use it in small quantities. I have frequently come across sportsmen, in particular weightlifters and body builders, who boast of eating up to one hundred tablets per day. This is a mistake. The amount of protein which has to be handled by the liver (since the liver has the task of synthesising protein) is high and it may be overburdened. In moderation, however, yeast can be a valuable food for the sportsman and sportswomen.

GINSENG

Ginseng has been used by the Chinese for over five thousand years and it has gained great respect as an Eastern medicine.

In essence there are two types of ginseng: panax ginseng and eleutherococcus (Siberian ginseng). Of these, the former is classed as true ginseng. Originating from Manchuria, it is cultivated in China, Korea, Russia and Japan. Eleutherococcus, whilst strictly speaking botanically identical, is usually classified as part of the ginseng family because it has almost identical effects.

Ginseng is known as an adaptogen because it helps to normalise bodily functions when disharmony exists.

Ginseng, as an aid to the athlete is worthy of note because it is now established that it improves stamina and resistance to fatigue and stress. I would, therefore, suggest that further advice concerning this valuable product in terms of what to choose and how much to take, be sought from your nearest health food store. It is worth noting, however, that when taking ginseng, you should avoid other stimulants such as tea, coffee and cola drinks. Women should not take it when pregnant, breast feeding, or when suffering from breast cancer, unless under medical supervision.

THE ANTI-OXIDANT NUTRIENTS

Anti-oxidants are fast gaining a reputation as protective factors that come to the body's defence against the effects of pollution and stress. Unfortunately, we live in a world in which we are all subjected to exposure to unnatural chemicals of all kinds, such as car exhaust fumes, pesticides and other agricultural chemicals. These pollutants, once inside the body, can cause the over-production of free radicals, which are highly destructive unstable molecules which can attack the body's cells, resulting in oxidation damage. In simple terms, fat in the cells goes rancid, as would butter left out in the sun. Accumulating evidence from around the world strongly indicates that such free radical damage is connected with heart disease, premature ageing and cancer.

The antioxidant nutrients have been observed to neutralise free radicals, thus preventing their harmful effects. In addition, some of these nutrients have been linked with improving performance as a result of their ability to enhance the body's utilisation of oxygen. Vitamin E, in particular, is often used by sports people when great cardiovascular demands are placed upon the body, for example in sprinting or long-distance running.

Interestingly enough, an increasing number of athletes are now taking anti-oxidant nutrients to help protect them against air pollution. When we consider that an athlete training outside can use up to twenty times more oxygen than the average person out for a walk, it may well be a sensible precaution to ensure that the diet contains an ample amount of such nutrients.

In addition to vitamin E, the other main anti-oxidant nutrients are beta carotene, vitamin C and selenium, although new ones such as lycopene - found in tomatoes and thought to provide protection against prostate cancer - are constantly being identified. The thing to remember, however, is that these nutrients work synergistically, or as a team. Therefore, it is wise to take a combination formula which contains the full spectrum of these nutrients in their correct balance. Once again, further information can be derived either from the library or health food store.

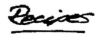

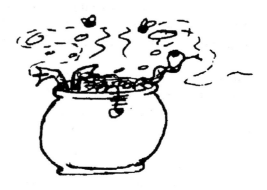

CHAPTER 4   **RECIPES**

The following recipes are intended to serve as examples of ways in which some of the aforementioned fitness foods can be utilised by those engaged in sport. Try them and experiment where necessary, but remember that a whole new field of discovery is open to you.

Honey And Milk Energy Booster
As a pre-competition drink the honey and milk formula can be recommended (unless you are one of those unfortunate people who are allergic to cow's milk, in which case try switching to goat's milk). This formula is particularly suitable to the sports participant on two counts: 1) It provides a source of quick energy in the form of simple sugars present in the honey. 2) It has a sustaining effect, which can be attributed to the lactose in milk (another sugar). Lactose, unlike the simple sugars present in the honey is of the complex variety and subsequently has to be broken down by the digestive system - this takes time, and thus the energy available to the body from the lactose is provided after some delay. The end result of this process is a supply of both short and long term energy - the former from the honey, and the latter from the milk. In addition, the milk provides us with protein (approximately fifteen grammes), and fat for long term sustenance; although with regard to the latter, it is best to use milk that is lower in fat such as semi-skimmed.

It is well known that such pursuits as tennis, soccer, hockey, basketball, long distance running and swimming, create heavy demands on the body, therefore, the honey and milk combination may be worth trying.

I suggest that you drink an average size glass of the honey and milk mixture no later than twenty five minutes before a match or event. I would recommend that you opt for organic milk, since this will be free from antibiotics, agricultural chemicals and hormones etc.

Method Of Preparation
Put into a liquidiser or mixing bowl the following ingredients:
1. Half a pint of milk (preferably unpasteurised goat's milk).
2. One tablespoonsful of honey.
Simply mix the two ingredients using a liquidiser or hand whisk until perfectly blended.

* Goat's milk, if unpasteurised, is much to be preferred to cow's milk since it is easily digested and less mucus-forming. In addition, if you suffer from sinus problems, try cutting out dairy products, with the exception of unpasteurised goat's milk and yoghurt. Unpasturised goat's milk is becoming more difficult to find due to legislation concerning bacterial contamination. You will need to use your own judgement in terms of what you select. Personally, I've been drinking unpasteurised goat's milk for many years with no problems.

High Protein
The following recipe makes a good high protein drink ideal as a protein supplement and particularly beneficial to men and women who have to meet the body's requirements for protein as a result of muscular wear and tear.

Method
Take a dessertspoonful of whey powder, a dessertspoonful of powdered brewer's yeast and three-quarters of a glass of water. Make up the

mixture with a fruit juice of your choice such as apple, pineapple or orange (the pure unsweetened variety). Mix well and drink chilled if desired. Pineapple juice is particularly beneficial because it contains the protein-digesting enzyme BROMELAIN.

Weight Watcher's Sustainer
This is useful as a sustaining drink to the weight conscious person who is engaged in sport and wishes to avoid putting on superfluous weight.

Method
Add a tablespoon of powdered brewer's yeast to a glass of chilled grapefruit, apple or orange juice, mix thoroughly.

Fruit And Yoghurt Delight
Combines the health-giving properties of fruit and yoghurt in a palatable form.

Method
Simply liquidise a quantity of soft fruit such as pears or melon, until a puree is produced, add yoghurt, sprinkle some chopped nuts or wheatgerm on top of the mixture and add a little honey to sweeten if necessary.

Molasses Milk Shake
An extremely palatable method of consuming molasses is to take it in the form of a milk shake. This counteracts its slightly bitter taste.

Method
Place half a pint of skimmed milk into a liquidiser or mixing bowl, add approximately one tablespoon of molasses and liquidise until frothy, drink immediately before the mixture separates.

Breakfast Special
For a health-giving breakfast using the following natural foods use the following method:
Take one dessertspoonful of honey, add this to some yoghurt, mix well, then add a sprinkling of wheatgerm or chopped nuts. If desired, substitute molasses or black treacle for honey.

Health Salad
It is always a good idea to have at least one large salad a day. This needn't consist of the traditional boring lettuce leaf, boiled egg and cucumber, etc. The number of interesting healthy salad dishes are almost infinite. For instance, consider the following combinations:

Coleslaw
This consists of thinly shredded carrot and white cabbage, perhaps with finely sliced onion too. Raisins and nuts can also be added. Unless you wish to make your own salad dressing, I would suggest that you purchase some of the really good healthy brands currently available from health food stores. Most of these are made from cider vinegar, which is far better for you compared to other vinegars.

Finger Salad
Bits of raw cauliflower, slices of green and red peppers, carrot sticks, spring onions, cherry tomatoes and celery served with a nice chilled dressing or favourite dip.

Brown Rice Salad
Brown rice, toasted peanuts, diced green and red peppers, broad beans or peas, and a cider vinegar and oil dressing (one part vinegar to two parts oil).

Bean Salad
Lightly cooked green beans and cooked beans of your choice (example haricot); add chunks of celery, onions, etc., and a suitable dressing.

Niçoise
Quartered tomatoes, black olives, lightly cooked green beans, anchovies, hard boiled egg in quarters, and tuna fish. Add a suitable dressing.

Caesar Salad
Pieces of crisp lettuce, parmesan cheese and chopped poached or scrambled egg (preferably free range). Croutons made from wholemeal bread (simply fry in oil flavoured with crushed garlic), add a suitable dressing.

Mixed Salad
Mix in a large salad bowl whatever combinations of salad and fruit ingredients desired: example, dates, raisins, lettuce, onions, radish, apple, cabbage, tomatoes, cauliflower, carrots, nuts, cucumber, cheese pieces (or substitute organic/GMO free tofu, a soya bean curd); add favourite dressing. The advantage of this type of salad is that it can be stored in the refrigerator and eaten when required, preferably within twenty-four hours.

Obviously the foregoing recipe suggestions are merely examples. Even if you discover that not one of them appeals to your palate, this should not deter you from trying other ideas. Remember there is a whole new world of foods for you to explore. All that is required is a little patience and the willingness to experiment in order to discover what suits you best. As stated earlier, the path that leads us to improved health and fitness is seldom an easy one, being lined with obstacles and temptations that will lead you in the wrong direction. Nevertheless, it may be worth remembering that everything worth achieving has to be worked for. Seldom do we get anything for nothing, and this applies no less when striving to improve one's health and well-being.

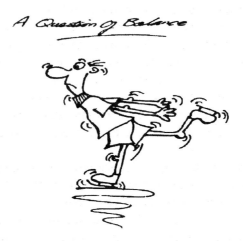

A Question of Balance

CHAPTER 5   A QUESTION OF BALANCE

From Palaeolithic times until quite recently, people have lived close to nature. In fact, the modern athlete would look pretty tame in comparison to some of our muscular, spear-wielding ancestors, who had to rely on their natural physical and mental abilities in order to survive.

Even today, it has been reported by learned observers of primitive tribes in such regions as South America and Australia, that the sheer athletic ability of some of these people is quite astounding.

The aborigine, for example, was a born hunter before the advent of modernisation. Often his only weapon was a crudely manufactured spear, but before this could be used, he had to get close enough to his prey. This would often involve a full-blooded chase for many miles without rest. How many top athletes, let alone average members of the public, could match up to this kind of physical endeavour?

It is also significant that the commonly accepted diseases of modern society, such as cancer, diabetes, heart disease and high blood pressure, are virtually unknown to many primitive people who live a more natural lifestyle. It is only when these primitive races are introduced to our modern diet, as has happened in the past, that they begin to suffer from the same aforementioned diseases. For instance, the people of Hunza, a small isolated country near Pakistan, were renowned for their tremendous health, longevity and freedom from disease. Sadly, these people were soon to develop the common afflictions of the western world, but only after civilisation eventually broke through to them.

A major aspect of the original Hunza diet was its inherent balance between alkaline-forming and acid-forming foods. This was partly dictated by the environment, that is, what foods were available, however, it would appear that these people had an almost innate understanding that a healthy diet should be predominantly alkaline-forming. Certainly with the emphasis on wild apricots and other fruits and vegetables, the Hunzas were adhering to a diet which is highly recommended by most nutritionists and naturopaths today.

Getting The Balance Right

The planning of a diet which is designed to promote health and well-being, and thus lay open a channel that will lead the body towards overall improved fitness, must of necessity, not merely concern itself with the wise and judicious choice of natural foods, but also in the body's acid\alkaline balance.

The emphasis must be placed upon selecting foods which are predominately alkaline-forming. Broadly speaking, the overall balance should comprise of:

70/75% fruit and vegetables - since these foods are the chief alkaline foods, they must figure as the prominent part of the diet.

25/30% nuts, bread, meat, cheese, cereals, pulses etc, as these represent the principle acid-forming foods.

A balanced diet, therefore, would consist of the following proportions:

PROTEIN - (15%)   Cottage cheese, mushrooms, almonds, peanuts, walnuts, eggs, pulses, meat (preferably from naturally reared animals) and fish

CARBOHYDRATES (15%)   100% wholewheat flour (preferably stoneground and organically grown), other wholegrain cereals such as corn, rye and oats, wholegrain pasta and rice, honey and molasses.

FATS - (5%)   Butter (in moderation), vegetable margarine (select a product which is made from natural ingredients and that is unhydrogenated), sunflower, safflower and other seed oils.

FRUIT AND VEG.(65%)   Fruits of all kinds with half eaten in their natural raw state.

Serious and not so serious sports participants would do well to base their diet on the foregoing proportions. In this way, such a diet will fulfil the following functions:

a)   Supply a low cholesterol and high alkaline diet.
b)   Provide the body with an ample supply of vitamins and minerals in their natural balance, since they are being supplied to the body as nature intended.

c)   Significantly reduce the intake of chemical additives often present in de-natured and refined foods.
d)   Provide an abundance of fibre which is now recognised as being important in preventing a number of diseases such as cancer of the colon.

To further facilitate the planning of a healthy diet I have included here some examples of acid-forming and alkaline-forming foods:

Acid-forming
Meat, fish, nuts, honey, bread, cereals, legumes (eg: peas, beans, lentils), rice, seeds, (e.g. sunflower and sesame), most cheeses except cottage.

Alkaline-forming
Fruits (e.g. Pears, apples, pineapples, grapes, oranges, papayas etc.)
Dried fruits such as raisins, sultanas and figs (purchase only preservative free fruit, preferably organically grown).
Vegetables: e.g. turnips, beetroot, tomatoes, cabbage, carrots, potatoes (usually cooked in their skins to preserve their nutrients). Liquids - unsweetened fruit juices such as apple, pear, grape and orange.

Having given you some of the basic ingredients of a wholefood diet, let us see how these may be arranged in the form of a menu:

BREAKFAST: choose one or more of the following:

1.   Fresh fruit juice.
2.   Muesli with fresh fruit.
3.   Yoghurt (select only natural yoghurt which is free from additives and sugar. Sweeten if desired with a little honey or dark-brown sugar.)
4.   Soaked dried fruit with wheatgerm if desired.

MID-DAY:

1. One large salad of fresh green or root vegetables. Experiment with a variety of dressings available from the health food store, or try your own using such ingredients as cider vinegar, lemon juice and olive oil. (some organic ready made dressings are now available from health food shops and supermarkets.)
2. Grated cheese or nuts.
3. Wholewheat bread or crispbread with a little butter or margarine.

EVENING MEAL: choose from

1. Home-made soup or salad.
2. A savoury protein dish.
3. Vegetables, steamed or conservatively cooked with little water.
4. Jacket potato stuffed with cheese or onions, parsnips, tomatoes, etc.

DESSERT: choose from

1. Fresh or dried fruit.
2. Yoghurt.
3. Home-made egg custard or natural jelly (available from health food stores).
4. Natural soya dessert made from organic/GMO free soya.
5. Organic ice-cream.

When purchasing food, it is always worth seeking out organically grown produce, since this is free from agricultural chemicals such as artificial nitrates and pesticides, which may actually negate your efforts to achieve improved health and efficiency. The very fact that we are unaware of their potential harmful effects should act as a warning signal to most people who are clued in to the benefits of a natural lifestyle.

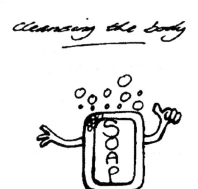

Cleansing the body

CHAPTER 6   CLEANSING THE BODY

There are a variety of methods that we can employ in order to rid the body of harmful toxins. These toxic accumulations are often linked with feeling under-par; they are sometimes responsible for a whole host of bodily ailments such as migraines, digestive complaints, frequent colds and other infections, and, as I discovered for myself, at least some forms of arthritis and other rheumatic complaints. When the level of toxicity is allowed to build up, often over a period of years, then more serious diseases may manifest themselves in the body.

Even a seemingly healthy person can benefit from a thorough cleansing, and this is no less true for those engaged in sport. In fact, it is not at all unusual for sportsmen and women to experience a general feeling of improved well-being after following a cleansing regime, and of course this may result in improved performance.

The objective is to eliminate harmful toxic elements from the body, to restore efficient metabolic functioning and to prepare oneself for a natural, wholesome diet.

The All Fruit Diet

As I stated earlier in this book, fruit and vegetables are excellent medicines as well as superior foods. Because they have a cleansing effect in the body, fruit and vegetables will eliminate toxins most effectively when consumed in the form of a temporary mono-diet.

All fruits and vegetables are suitable, except potatoes and bananas, which have a high starch content, and will hamper the cleansing process.

Some authorities are of the opinion that fruit and vegetables should be eaten separately, as they conflict with each other in the process of their digestion. It may, therefore, be worth giving this approach a try. For example, by having an all-fruit meal for lunch and an all vegetable meal for the evening meal. Since this diet is to be adhered to for perhaps a week or two, it may not be too arduous to follow, especially when one considers the improvement that often ensues after sticking to this limited regime.

When employing this approach you would be wise to drink only unsweetened fruit juices such as apple. Furthermore, the consumption of purified water at such a time helps greatly in aiding the body to eliminate toxic waste that has been stored in the body, sometimes for a considerable period.

Fasting

Of all the methods used to cleanse the body of toxins, fasting is the quickest. I suggest that short, periodic fasts would be best, rather than lengthy fasts which may require the supervision of a trained practitioner. For instance, fasting for just a couple of days once or twice a month, with a longer fast of around a week, or once or twice a year, should produce good results. Naturally, care should be exercised when planning the timing of these fasts, taking care not to abstain from food when energy demands are great. Some people fast on purified water, or mineral water* only, others prefer to fast on fruit and vegetable juices, however, both methods are known to be efficacious.

When preparing to fast, it is important to eat just fruit and vegetables the day before; then, after the fast is over, say after two days, you should again consume only fruit and vegetables the day after. Gradually, over the next few days, you will be able to add other foods such as jacket potatoes and cottage cheese to the menu. This pre-fast and post-fast routine is very important if the value of the fast is not to be lost.

When in the process of fasting, take care not to be too energetic, however, light exercise is to be recommended with plenty of relaxation in between.

Cleansing Reactions
Whilst in the process of cleansing the system, do not be surprised if you experience some uncomfortable symptoms such as a coated tongue, headaches, dull eyes and a pallid complexion. The severity of these symptoms indicate the degree of toxicity of the body. In other words, the more toxic you are, the greater the discomfort.

The symptoms are actually a good sign in that they indicate that the body has started to clear out toxic waste which is then eliminated through the normal channels of excretion, namely, the kidneys, lungs, colon and skin. This should therefore not be misconstrued as something negative, but rather an encouraging sign. Nevertheless, should these toxins be eliminated too rapidly, then the normal excretory channels may become overburdened. This can be avoided if you use an enema or a suitable herbal preparation in order to aid in the elimination of toxic waste from the system. Do remember that you will have been accumulating toxins over many years and you shouldn't expect these to be expelled from your system with just one fast. However, with each successive fast you will be on course for achieving your overall objective - that of purifying your body and thus enhancing its physical condition.

*Purified water, which is free from all contaminants, is worth using for the purpose of fasting. Alternatively, you can use natural spring water, although personally I try to avoid water from areas which may have been affected by the Chernobyl disaster, such as certain parts of Scotland and Wales. Tap water is unsuitable because it contains too many contaminants such as fluoride, nitrates and heavy metals.

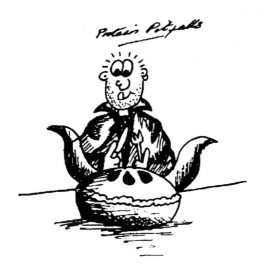

CHAPTER 7   **AVOIDING THE PROTEIN PITFALLS**

When I was a young man in my late teens I used to train with a fine bunch of men at the Sunderland Health and Strength Club, as it was then known. Very often the subject of diet as an aid towards improved results in sport, would creep into the conversation. In particular, the merits of good nutrition, especially for those who were aspiring towards building a more muscular physique, would be the focus for our attention.

Unfortunately, most of the body builders in that club had jumped on the 'protein bandwagon', including, I have to say, myself at one stage. Admittedly, an increase in muscular size and strength ensued as a result of the combination of dedicated training and a high protein diet; but not, as it transpired, without a price to pay. I soon began to realise from my own experience and observations, that too much protein could be an enemy as well as an aid. This was brought home to me in no uncertain terms when I observed the number of bodybuilders who succumbed to colds and 'flu, often after making great progress after several weeks of hard training.

I soon came to the conclusion that excess protein in the diet was their problem. This in turn resulted in the production of too much uric acid in the body, since this is the end-product of protein digestion. I soon began to notice in my own case that too much protein resulted in a greater susceptibility to colds, 'flu and other infections. To me, this was further evidence of the intricate link between diet and illness, and it made me think, even in those early days, of the possible far-reaching effects of diet on athletic performance.

Interestingly enough, many years after reaching this conclusion, I engaged myself in a personal experiment, the results of which may have widespread implications. Being now in my forties, my weight training endeavours have levelled out a little, preferring as I do to participate in fast action sports such as five-a-side football, which has always been a love of mine. Nevertheless, having joined a new gym near my home town, I set about training with renewed enthusiasm. It was whilst engaged in this training that I decided to follow a fruit and vegetable diet in order to give my system a 'houseclean', which is something that I do on a periodic basis so that harmful toxins can be eliminated. To be perfectly frank I was anticipating a significant reduction in my strength capacity, since at one time I was consuming no complete protein at all for over two weeks. You can imagine my surprise, therefore, when I discovered that my strength was not declining, but actually increasing, and that I still had lots of energy into the bargain. Of course, this state of affairs would not have been maintained on such a cleansing diet, since protein is required to replace muscle tissue. However, it made me acutely aware that it was possible to do well on far less protein than is commonly accepted. This is not to say that there are no fluctuations in protein requirements from individual to individual, but that personal experimentation with protein needs and performance may be beneficial in this regard.

Furthermore, whilst acknowledging that some sports people, because of the physical demands of their sport, do require more protein than others (such as weightlifters and shot putters), it may be worth bearing in mind that if an above-average protein intake is adhered to, then a subsequent increase in fruit and vegetables should follow, since this will help to neutralise any excess acid in the system.

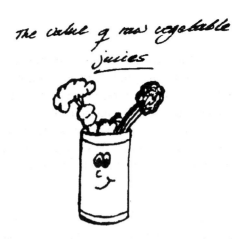

The value of raw vegetable juices

CHAPTER 8   THE VALUE OF RAW VEGETABLE JUICES

Raw vegetable juices are an excellent source of vitamins, minerals and enzymes. Also, since they are generally alkaline-forming, they can enhance a diet which is based upon the naturopathic principles already outlined.

The key to nourishing your body is the 'life force' which is present in the foods that we consume. Our bodies are made up of millions of microscopic living units called cells. These cells require a good supply of nutrients in the correct proportions in order to function properly, and replenish themselves. This process of cell regeneration cannot continue efficiently if we are in the habit of consuming 'lifeless' foods such as white sugar, white flour, chocolate bars and canned drinks. This is because these foods are lacking in such factors as vitamins and enzymes which are essential if proper nourishment is to take place. If we base our diet on 'living' foods such as raw vegetables and fruits, we are providing ourselves with the finest kind of nourishment that nature can provide.

One method of furnishing our cells with a generous supply of health-giving nutrients, is to get into the daily habit of drinking raw vegetable juices. Some people will no doubt ask the question: 'Why don't we just eat the whole vegetables and be done with it?' The answer is quite straightforward, in that raw solid food requires a lot of digestion, sometimes over several hours, before its nourishment can be used by the cells. This is because raw food contains an abundance of fibre. Therefore, by removing the fibre, nutrients from the juices are much more readily available. Imagine, for example, eating your way through a pound of carrots, and contrast this with drinking a glass of carrot juice. The advantages then become immediately obvious.

Juice Preparation

In order to prepare your own juices you will need to invest in a juice extractor. There are two basic types: the centrifugal extractor, which as the name suggests, works on the principle of centrifugal force, and the juice press.

Of the two, the latter is the best from a nutritional point of view, since the pressing method extracts juice without exposing it to as much air as the centrifugal method. Such exposure to air results in a greater loss of nutrients, especially enzymes which are very important for our health. Unfortunately, the pressing method tends to be more time consuming and somewhat messy. The majority of people, therefore, tend to use the centrifugal type of extractor; especially as the food value of the resulting juice is far from lost. It is worth remembering, however, that freshly prepared juices need to be either drunk immediately, or refrigerated for no more than a few hours before consumption. This is important since the 'living' qualities of the juice will begin to deteriorate once the juices are separated from the cells of the plant from which they originate.

How Much Juice Should We Drink?

Generally speaking, one should drink at least one pint of juice daily, this being a minimum quantity if results are to show themselves. However, two to eight pints will usually be more productive, particularly when accompanied by a balanced wholefood diet.

Types of juices

Raw Carrot

This is the richest source of beta carotene which is converted by the body into vitamin A. Vegetables which contain an abundance of this vitamin are now being recommended as a cancer preventative, because recent studies have revealed that there may be a connection between an ample supply of this nutrient in the diet and at least some cancers.

Carrots also contain a good supply of vitamins B, C, D, E, G and K. They possess powerful cleansing properties, particularly where the liver is concerned; and for this reason, it is perhaps wise to gradually increase the quantity consumed.

Carrot juice is also said to strengthen the lungs, largely because of its beta carotene content. Furthermore, it aids the body in resisting infections.

You may find that your skin takes on a distinct orange colour, a condition which shows itself when you have been drinking carrot juice regularly. If this happens, do not concern yourself, since it is a perfectly harmless indication that the juice is giving your liver a much needed cleansing. Carrot juice also contains an abundant supply of minerals, such as sodium, potassium, calcium, iron, and magnesium.

Beet Juice

This is another extremely valuable juice which also has a powerful cleansing effect. For this reason, do not drink more than a wineglassful at a time, if taken by itself. More of the juice can be taken if it is added to other juices such as carrot and celery.

Beet juice is rich in valuable nutrients and it is especially valued for its blood building qualities, in that it nourishes the red blood corpuscles and has a general blood toning effect. There is also evidence that suggests that beetroot and its juice possesses anti-cancer properties.

For this reason it is often included in diets designed to help cure cancer, along with carrot juice, since together they have a potent effect.

Celery Juice
This contains an exceptional amount of organic sodium, an element which is extremely good for arthritis sufferers. Sodium is important in maintaining the normal physiological processes of the body, in particular, the fluidity of the blood and lymph.

Celery is also rich in other organic minerals including magnesium, calcium and iron; all of which are easily assimilated by the body. In fact, drinking such raw juices as celery and carrot as a source of organic minerals and vitamins, is far preferable than taking them artificially in the form of tablets, as the body cannot assimilate them to the same extent.

Cucumber Juice
Cucumber acts as a natural diuretic and bodybuilders who are attempting to gain greater definition by cutting down on liquid intake prior to competition, would be far better advised to use cucumber for its diuretic properties, than resort to harmful drugs.

Cucumber juice is high in potassium, sodium, chlorine, calcium, silicon and sulphur. It is good in combination with beetroot, carrot and lettuce, as a body cleanser. Its high potassium content makes it a good alkaline-forming juice as well as being helpful in improving low and high blood pressure.

Cucumber juice is also said to be good for the skin, nails and hair, especially when combined with carrot and lettuce juice.

Lettuce Juice
The body is in constant need of an adequate supply of iron and it is stored in the liver and spleen to be used as a reserve when extra iron is called for, for example, after the loss of blood. Lettuce juice is to be

highly valued, therefore, since it is very rich in iron. Lettuce also contains a good supply of magnesium, a necessary component in regeneration of cells, particularly in relation to the cells of the lungs and nerves.

A good combination for lettuce juice is that of carrot because the organic constituents of both are extremely compatible.

Green Pepper Juice
This juice is rich in vitamin C which is important in the prevention of infections and in the repair of the body's connective tissues. Pepper juice is rich in silicon, which makes it good for skin, nails and hair.

It is good in combination with carrot in the proportion of half green pepper juice and half carrot.

Potato Juice
Raw potato juice is rich in organic phosphorous, potassium, sulphur and chlorine. When the potato is cooked these atoms are converted into inorganic atoms, and as such are not so easily used by the body.

Raw potato juice is an excellent cleanser and for this reason is to be recommended for those who suffer from arthritis. Always select organic potatoes, however, and avoid using those that are green, as these are high in a poison called solanine.

Spinach Juice
Spinach juice is highly recommended for the digestive tract. It has the ability to cleanse and regenerate the entire colon. Spinach juice, amongst other things, is also very good for bleeding gums, particularly when in combination with carrot juice.

Spinach has a high oxalic acid content which explains its laxative properties. However, when it is eaten cooked, the oxalic acid can form crystals in our kidneys resulting in kidney trouble.

Tomato Juice

This has a good cleansing effect, and is thus beneficial; however, this only applies when it is consumed in the absence of concentrated starches, such as bread and cereals.

Tomato juice is rich in magnesium, potassium, sodium and calcium, and when fresh, it has a good vitamin C content.

Of course, there are many other juices that are beneficial for their health-giving and healing properties. With regard to the latter, specific combinations of juices are useful as a means of eradicating a variety of illnesses. I would suggest, therefore, that it would be worthwhile seeking books from the health food store or the library which deal with the fascinating subject of raw juices and their properties in great detail. In essence, however, it can be clearly determined that raw vegetable juices can form an extremely valuable component of a natural lifestyle. An observation which needs to be considered carefully by all those involved in sport; especially those who wish to improve performance, increase longevity, prolong an active lifestyle and build a strong resistance to disease.

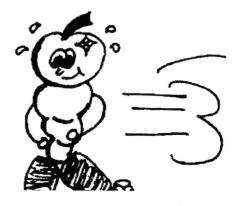

vegetarian athlete

CHAPTER 9   THE VEGETARIAN ATHLETE

Even today, in this increasingly enlightened age, it is surprising that so many people remain under the delusion that meat is good for you. The myth that it is an almost essential component of the sportsman's and sportswoman's diet, still lingers on. Nevertheless, an increasing number of athletes are now becoming aware that meat is not only not essential, it is not even necessary. Many vegetarian athletes will now testify to this, particularly those in the very top flight of sport who are amongst our finest athletes.

One offshoot of this slow change in attitude is the switch from the traditional steak as a pre-match meal, to the high carbohydrate meal, such as pasta or spaghetti, which are recognised as providing long-term energy. This was very much in evidence during the last World Cup football competition, when the England team were seen happily tucking into plates of pasta and spaghetti, and what's more, being encouraged to do so.

But why has this change of attitude towards meat occurred? At one time meat was valued for its strength-giving properties; however, more people are becoming aware that meat, far from enhancing health and strength, is actually very hard to digest and produces harmful toxins, which then have to be dealt with by the body. Naturally meat is a high protein food, but other foods provide equal amounts of protein and don't have the same disadvantages. Vegetable proteins derived from pulses, nuts and in particular the versatile soya bean, although classed as second class proteins, when mixed, provide the full spectrum of amino-acids that are necessary for tissue replacement. This includes the physiological processes in the body that require protein; for example, digestion of food requires a variety of enzymes, which are made from protein.

Vegetable proteins possess several advantages over animal proteins. They are less acid-forming, more easily digested, and perhaps most important of all, do not produce toxic waste products in the way that meat does during the process of digestion. In this context, some nutritionists and health practitioners regard second class proteins as first class; and first class proteins are relegated to the position of second class proteins.

Certainly, when we observe the people of the world who have a reputation for good health and longevity, such as the Vilcabamba in Ecuador and the Abkhazians, formerly of the Soviet Republic of Georgia, it becomes obvious that their diets consist principally of vegetable proteins, and sometimes a small amount of animal protein such as unpasteurised milk, yoghurt, or a little meat. This is also consistent with the observations made by Sir Robert McCarrison on the Hunza people in the early part of this century.

Obviously the decision of whether to include meat in your daily diet lies with the reader, but if you are to include it, try to select mainly white meat, such as that from chicken; and if you can find a supply of naturally reared, additive free meat, then this is preferable to commercially reared produce, especially bearing in mind the controversy surrounding beef products and their safety.

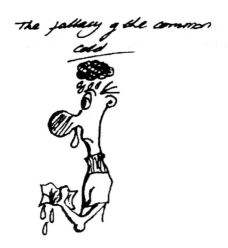

The fallacy of the common cold

CHAPTER 10   THE FALLACY OF THE COMMON COLD

Many years ago, when I discovered a natural approach for my arthritis, I was amazed to learn that naturopathic and other alternative medical practitioners, did not subscribe to the theory that the common cold is caused by germs. Instead, the idea that a cold is merely the body's way of eliminating harmful toxins in the form of mucus, forms the foundation of the natural approach.

This, admittedly, was somewhat hard to swallow. After all, are we not all brought up to believe passionately in the germ theory, as expounded by that eminent scientist Pasteur himself? How else could colds be transferred from person to person? It had to be those malevolent microbes! And yet, years of personal experience has since confirmed to me the validity of the naturopathic interpretation behind the origin of colds. Certainly, if the mucus of the cold sufferer is scrutinised under a microscope, germs will indeed be isolated. Nevertheless, these germs would appear not to be the cause of the illness, but merely a manifestation of it. Put simply, these seemingly hostile germs are nature's scavengers, proliferating on the toxic laden mucus that is expelled from our bodies, feeding on it, as do microbes on a decomposing piece of meat. They do not cause the symptoms of ill health that accompany a cold; the elimination of toxic waste from the body brings this about.

This is why a cold, handled correctly, is actually a positive process, since it acts as nature's safety valve when the toxins in the body reach saturation point. Unfortunately, instead of aiding nature in her elimination of toxins, by drinking juices and fasting for a day or two, what do we do? Why, we compound the problem by taking medicinal preparations such as pain-killers, cough medicines and decongestants, in order to alleviate the symptoms. This of course is merely forcing even more toxins back into the system, with the consequence of more serious illnesses developing in the future.

Speaking from personal experience, I know that if I go on a food binge, which, being only human, I occasionally do: then, after a while, not only do my arthritic symptoms begin to rear their ugly head, but I will often develop a cold. Sometimes this will happen when I revert back to a cleansing diet, and it has led me to believe that toxins that have accumulated as a result of my dietary indiscretions, are being eliminated when my body is suddenly switched to a 'cleansing mode'. If you like, it appears that I am actually capable of self-inducing a cold in this way. Conversely, I have learned over the years, that when I adhere to a wholesome, alkaline-forming diet, then it is extremely rare for me to develop a cold, or any other infection, even though I am often constantly exposed to sneezes and coughs from the staff and pupils around me.

The next time that you develop a cold, therefore, attempt to aid your body in eliminating its toxic waste, and try regarding the cold as nature's warning signal, telling you that your system requires a good 'housecleaning'. To suppress a cold with drugs or junk food, only invites future health problems.

This is not to suggest that I am against medication when it is absolutely necessary, for example, the use of antibiotics may be a lifesaver in certain situations. However, if a natural lifestyle is adhered to, the need for such medication should decrease in proportion to the purity of the body. What's more, the body's immune system will be able to function more efficiently, being less encumbered by an unbalanced diet and the many chemicals which most people consume on a regular basis. My advice, therefore, would be to avoid the mistake of adopting a purist approach concerning the use of medication when it is absolutely necessary. When the condition has cleared up, you can always revert back to a cleansing diet in order to build up your immune system.

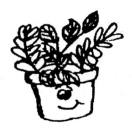

CHAPTER 11   **PLANT POWER - HERBS;
THE ATHLETE'S ALLY**

Herbs have been used for centuries as a source of food and medicine for mankind. Our ancestors accumulated a vast wealth of knowledge concerning the medicinal properties of herbs and many volumes have since been written on the subject. What is particularly exciting, in view of earlier scepticism from orthodox doctors, is the increasing impressive evidence from modern scientific studies which have helped to validate the claims by herbalists concerning specific plants and their medicinal properties. A good example concerns comfrey, a herb which was referred to by herbalists as 'knitbone' due to its reputation as a healer of broken bones.

Fairly recent research into this plant resulted in the isolation of a chemical called allantoin, which is an important component of comfrey. Significantly, allantoin is now known to influence the reproduction of bone cells thus speeding up repair to breaks and fractures. Comfrey ointment can now be purchased from the health food shops and some chemists. Applied externally it is used to help heal injuries, which is a useful aid to all those involved in sport.

Research into the healing and protective properties of plants has never been as intense as it is today and every day we seem to hear about a new and exciting discovery. In the light of this fact, many people are now turning to natural remedies as an answer to their health problems and as an important part of a healthier lifestyle.

It is heartening to hear that top athletes are now beginning to explore the possibility of using certain herbs in order to enhance performance and help them increase their resistance to illness. In fact, staying free from illness, as many athletes will testify, is of vital importance because, apart from injury, ill health is the biggest threat to training and participation in competitions.

Bearing this in mind therefore, I have endeavoured to include in this chapter some examples of herbs which I consider to be a useful addition to the dietary changes we have already addressed earlier in this book.

Echinacea

Sometimes referred to as the purple cone flower because of its cone-shaped flowers, this herb has several valuable properties. Used originally by the American Indians who recognised its ability to help heal wounds, it is known to strengthen the body's immune system, thus increasing our resistance to infections such as colds and flu. One of the reasons for this is that it has been shown to actually increase the body's white blood cell count. This in turn helps us to resist infections, since white blood cells represent one of the body's major defences against harmful organisms.

Furthermore, echinacea does possess natural antiviral and antibacterial properties and used in conjunction with other immune-enhancing herbs, it is a valuable supplement which can be introduced into the daily dietary regime.

How it is taken
Echinacea can be taken in the form of tablets or as a herbal tincture. The latter is probably more effective since it comes in the form of a

liquid and can be taken by adding the appropriate number of drops to water or fruit juice. Also, being in liquid form it is more readily absorbed into the bloodstream. Ask your local health food store for brands that have a good reputation for quality.

Aloe Vera
This plant is a member of the lily and onion family and it is also related to asparagus and garlic. There are more than 300 varieties of aloe vera, but only a few are known to possess medicinal properties.

Aloe vera has been used by mankind for centuries as evidenced by references to the plant by the ancient Egyptians and several other cultures such as the Chinese and Indian peoples.

Aloe vera can be drunk as a nutritious health drink or a tonic and it can also be applied topically to the scalp and the skin as a lotion, cream or gel. There are some people who claim that aloe vera is a panacea for all ills. Personally I am very wary of such claims. Nevertheless, there is a wealth of medical evidence to suggest that aloe vera is effective in its positive influence on two areas of the body, namely the immune system and the epithelial tissue.

Epithelial tissue simply means a layer of cells that cover the surface of the body, such as the skin (the largest of our body organs) and internal surfaces such as the lining of the mouth, genitals, gastrointestinal tract, etc. Since aloe vera has a reputation as a healer of burns, and of skin conditions such as eczema, it is hardly surprising it can just as easily exert a healing influence on mouth ulcers, stomach ulcers or bowel problems, since these areas of the body, as already stated, comprise of epithelial tissue.

For those engaged in a lot of outdoor sport such as track and field athletics, when lots of sun exposure can be a problem, aloe vera can be used as an effective antidote to sunburn. Ideally it should be used in conjunction with a good quality sunblock. Also, since lots of sun exposure is known to accelerate ageing of the skin, it is perhaps worth noting that aloe vera does seem to exert an anti-ageing effect on the skin. This it achieves in many ways.

Firstly it contains polysaccharides which act as moisturisers. Secondly, when absorbed into the skin, aloe is also known to stimulate the fibroblasts to reproduce more quickly. These all produce collagen and elastin fibres, hence the skin becomes more elastic and less wrinkled. This is why aloe vera is often added to cosmetics for its moisturising and youth-promoting effects.

Taken internally, the juice of the plant is known to help conditions that arise as a result of the immune system over-reacting to agents such as bacteria, viruses or pollen. It would appear that aloe vera, taken internally, can either enhance or retard immune response to such foreign substances, therefore acting as a kind of moderator of the immune system. This may be why good results have been reported by sufferers of asthma and arthritis. Certainly asthma appears to be an increasingly common condition amongst athletes these days, and in this respect, the daily use of aloe vera juice may be worthy of consideration.

Perhaps its most valuable property in terms of those who are engaged in sports may be that aloe vera can be used as an anti-inflammatory. This is because inflammation is a common problem at the sight of an injury such as a joint, for example.

How it is taken
Externally, aloe vera can be used in the form of a creme or gel. Taken internally it can be consumed as pure aloe vera juice. Once opened however, the bottle should be kept in the refrigerator. Be careful to select a good quality juice when purchasing this product. It should be cold pressed, extracted from organically grown plants, and made from the pure juice, not concentrates.

I tend to add it in small quantities to fruit juices such as apple, which I feel makes it much more palatable. Some people are quite happy to drink the juice neat, although it has a slightly tart flavour. It is also possible to buy it with natural flavouring already added, e.g. cranberry.

Peppermint

Peppermint is undoubtedly one of my favourite herbs and I always make a point of taking it with me on my travels. Many people like to use peppermint tea bags which can be used to make a refreshing tea. I prefer to use the pure oil of peppermint which can be conveniently added to fruit juice.

Peppermint contains a number of therapeutic substances such as cineol which has antimicrobial properties, and menthol which is an antiseptic. It also has a soothing effect on the digestive system, helping to dispel wind and ease feelings of nausea.

Peppermint has a beneficial effect on the circulation reducing pain in the extremities caused by poor blood flow. Moreover, it is also known to help reduce leg cramps, swollen legs and varicose veins. It is sometimes taken as a remedy for migraine headaches. In some cases, while not curing the migraine attack, it at least helps to reduce its severity and the frequency of attacks.

In terms of its usefulness for all those engaged in sporting activity, I would thoroughly recommend anyone to include peppermint in their natural first aid kit. Also it can be included as an everyday addition to the dietary programme.

How it is taken

Peppermint can be purchased in the form of a tea (eg. as tea bags), tablets, capsules, powder and as peppermint oil. Whilst it is good in all of these forms, I personally prefer to use the pure oil of peppermint since this has no additives and providing you are careful to keep the bottle air-tight, it will last a long time.

As a refreshing pick-me-up, try adding a drop to some fruit juice such as apple and drinking it slowly. It is very refreshing, particularly when prior to engaging in sporting activity.

Garlic

Throughout the centuries, garlic has been held in very high esteem by people from all around the world. It is part of the onion family but whilst possessing many of the therapeutic properties of onions it is much more potent. Herbalists often refer to garlic as a pungent herb that wards off or clears bacterial infections. During the First World War, garlic was highly revered by the Russian army for its ability to protect against infections, so much so that it was referred to as the Russian penicillin.

In addition to its antibacterial and antiviral properties, garlic has received much publicity in recent years for its ability to help reduce blood cholesterol and lower blood pressure. This is very significant when you consider that heart disease and diseases of the circulatory system represent two of the major health concerns of modern times. When we consider just how preventable these life-threatening diseases are in the light of what we know about diet and supplements then it would seem to make sense to incorporate this wonderful natural food and medicine into our everyday diet - assuming of course that as an individual you find it tolerable. It's really one of those foods that we either love or hate. Having said this however, it is now true to say that garlic can be taken in a variety of ways as described.

How it is taken

Garlic is best taken raw, as a salad ingredient for example. Taken in this manner, all of its natural properties remain unspoiled and are therefore more potent. Nevertheless, should this method of consumption prove unpalatable, garlic can also be taken in the form of tablets and capsules, otherwise referred to as garlic pearles. The capsules are probably the next best thing to raw garlic in terms of their medicinal effect, since they comprise of garlic oil encapsulated within a gelatin shell. For those of us who are still a little cautious when it comes to consuming gelatin in view of the BSE crisis, then vegetarian capsules may be the answer; these are becoming increasingly available these days.

Consistent with the advice given earlier in this book, I would always urge people to select a good quality supplement made by a reputable company. In this respect, it is best to seek advice from the health food shop staff, many of whom are qualified in nutrition.

PLANT AID - FIRST AID HERBAL REMEDIES

Comfrey oil
Apply immediately to any bruises and injuries such as sprains. Helps to relieve the pain and speed up healing.

Tincture of arnica
As above.

Bach Rescue Remedy
Used to counteract shock. Can be taken every few minutes if necessary.

Camomile flowers
Relieves nausea and sickness. Also used to counteract nervousness.

Ginger (powdered or in tablet form)
To ease flatulence and indigestion. Half a teaspoonful in a little hot water can be sipped slowly. Also used to help prevent travel sickness. Being a natural remedy it is preferred to drugs.

Chickweed ointment
Helps to heal wounds, good for burns and to apply to wasp and bee stings. Sometimes used to draw abscesses.

Lavender oil
Diluted with a pure vegetable oil such as almond, it can be applied to the temples to ease headaches. Useful as an insect repellent and worth bearing in mind when training outdoors.

Peppermint oil
One drop in a little warm water or added to fruit juice to help with heartburn, indigestion and trapped wind. Will sometimes ease headaches, including migraines.

Echinacea
Can help us to overcome infections more rapidly. Best taken as drops in the form of a tincture - six to eight drops every hour. Can be used in conjunction with vitamin C to help boost the immune system.

Echinacea cream
Useful for speeding up the healing process for wounds such as cuts.

Calendula cream
Good for soothing sore and irritated skin.

Oil of cloves
Very useful as an emergency treatment for toothache. Dab a little oil onto some cotton wool and place over the troublesome tooth. It doesn't taste pleasant but it acts as an analgesic to kill the pain and an antiseptic to destroy harmful germs.

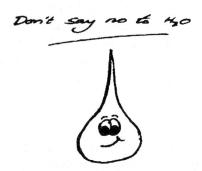

Don't say no to H₂O

CHAPTER 12   DON'T SAY NO TO H₂O! – AVOIDING THE RISKS OF DEHYDRATION

Although water is not classed as a nutrient, without it life would not exist. This is why human beings can survive for weeks without food, but only a matter of days without water. When we consider that around 60% of an adult's body weight consists of water, it is easy to see why it must be constantly replaced. This is especially important when we take into account that water is constantly being lost through breathing (about half a pint a day) and a considerable amount through sweating, depending on how much body heat you generate.

Water is important because:
- We need it for digestion - metabolic processes within the digestive system require water.
- Fluid in our blood is needed to transport nutrients, including energy-giving glucose to the muscles, and carry away metabolic by-products.
- Water is required in the production of urine so that waste products such as uric acid may be eliminated from the system.
- It acts as a lubricant in the body, e.g. for joints.
- It is essential in the regulation of body temperature.

Both food and drink supply water. Food roughly supplies a litre of fluid a day, although this may increase if the diet consists predominantly of fruit and vegetables. The rest is made up of drinks such as tea and coffee (I would recommend herbal teas and natural coffee substitutes) and juices. This makes up a total of around three litres of fluid each day.

Water and sport

When engaged in vigorous exercise, it is important that you drink more than normal. This can be achieved by drinking frequently prior to a training session or competitive situation. I would advise you to drink a large glass of pure water about ten minutes before commencing activity and to get into the habit of drinking regularly during drinks breaks, etc. Failure to do this could result in early fatigue, lack of concentration and headaches. This happens because the bodily wastes are not being dealt with effectively and as such, auto-intoxication will result.

These days many sports people choose so-called isotonic drinks which contain carbohydrate (for energy) and mineral salts. Having scrutinised the contents of some of these drinks, however, I have come to the conclusion that many contain dubious additives. A reasonable substitute would be a combination of unsweetened fruit juice (e.g. organic apple) and pure water. This provides both fluid and energy in a healthier way.

Foods with a high water content	% of water
cucumber	96
lettuce	96
melon	94
tomatoes	93
carrots	91
strawberries	89
peaches	86
oranges	86
apples	84
grapes	79
bananas	71

Once again, I must emphasise the importance of drinking plenty of water prior to sporting activity and also during activity when a break is possible (approximately every 15 minutes or so, although this could be increased in very hot conditions). Also, remember that when the activity is finished it is important to drink plenty of fluid to avoid dehydration.

The aim is to keep fluid levels up in order to avoid thirst, since when we are thirsty it is already an indication that fluid levels are not high enough.

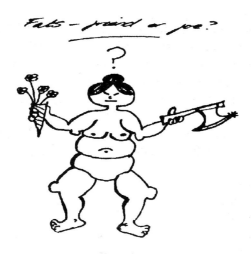

CHAPTER 13   FATS - FRIEND OR FOE?

Let's face it, fat has received a bad press over recent years, both in terms of its influence on obesity and its connection with cholesterol and heart disease. Unfortunately people are sometimes misled into believing that all fats are bad and this perception is reinforced by the emphasis currently being placed upon low fat foods in supermarkets and in television advertising.

The fact is that some fats are an essential part of our diet and without them we would not survive. Body fat is important for insulation and protection of the bodily organs. Some fat is stored around organs such as the liver, as an emergency energy supply in times of need. It is also a carrier for the fat-soluble vitamins such as A, E, D and K.

The problem for sports people and especially for more inactive members of the public, is that we only require a small amount of the essential fatty acids, or EFAs as they are called. But it is almost as if nature has set out to play a cruel joke on us, since so many tempting foods owe their flavour to the presence of fat. For example, we only need to think of cream cakes, chocolate, the wide diversity of cheeses, fried foods such as fish and chips, and meat roasts, to appreciate that temptation is all around us. Furthermore, to compound the problem, not all fat is so easily visible. It can be a hidden component of foods such as biscuits and nuts. Fat makes up a large proportion of nuts and when these are roasted, their fat content can markedly increase.

One of the main functions of fat is to supply us with energy, and weight for weight it has a little over twice the calories compared to carbohydrates and protein. Unfortunately, it is slow to be digested, which can be good for those involved with rigorous sport as long as the fatty food is consumed well in advance of the activity. This is why most nutritionists recommend sports people eat a high carbohydrate meal prior to a game or competition, since this is much more easily digested compared to a fatty meal.

Once digested, fat is broken down into fatty acids, cholesterol and phospholipids, the most recognised version of the latter being lecithin. The richest source of lecithin is egg yolks.

Fatty acids
There are over twenty fatty acids which form a natural component of fats. The two main types are:

Unsaturated fatty acids
Usually liquid at room temperature and come mainly from plants, e.g. sunflower and corn oil. However, they are also present in some fish and in chicken. Unsaturated fatty acids can be further divided into polyunsaturated (e.g. sunflower oil) and monounsaturated (olive and avocado oil). The body is capable of manufacturing all but three of the fatty acids, which is why these three are referred to as 'essential fatty acids', as shown below.

82

EFA	Source
Linoleic acid	derived from vegetable oils such as rapeseed and sunflower.
Linelenic acid	derived from fish such as herring and sardines.
Arachidonic acid	derived from beef, lamb, pork, liver and poultry.

Vegetarians can be reassured that arachidonic acid can be manufactured by the body from linoleic acid.

Omega 3

The essential fatty acids found in oily fish such as herring and mackerel. Current medical evidence suggests that if we increase our intake of Omega 3 fatty acids, then we are less likely to suffer from blood clots which can lead to heart attacks.

Saturated fatty acids

Usually solid at room temperature, they are derived largely from animal sources, such as meat, butter, cream and cheese. Surprisingly however, both coconut oil and palm oil are rich sources of saturated fats.

Cholesterol

Many people are under the misconception that all cholesterol is bad and should be kept to a minimum. However, cholesterol, which is present in all animal foods with the exception of egg white, is also manufactured by the body. This is because the body needs cholesterol as a component of body cells, blood and even hormones. It is also involved in the production of bile acids in the liver which help to absorb fats.

Nevertheless, it would appear that large amounts of cholesterol in the blood are associated with the onset of atherosclerosis or coronary heart disease - a condition brought about by fatty deposits clinging to the interior walls of blood vessels that lead to the heart, thus interfering with blood flow.

Unfortunately, the connection between dietary cholesterol and cholesterol in the blood is far from black and white, since some people develop high levels of cholesterol in their blood, despite the fact that they adhere to a low cholesterol diet.

There are two types of blood cholesterol, referred to as HDL (high density lipoproteins) and LDL (low density lipoproteins). Of the two, HDL is thought to be beneficial because it is believed to carry fats implicated in clogging arteries to the liver for disposal; whilst LDL is believed to encourage fatty deposits. It would appear, therefore, that our diets should contain high levels of HDL in order to discourage cholesterol build up in the arteries.

If all of this sounds as complicated as your average whodunit mystery, the plot is yet to reveal another twist, since, whilst saturated fats clearly increase levels of LDL and polyunsaturated fats seem to lower cholesterol, unfortunately this also means that beneficial HDL is lowered as well as the LDL (which we want to reduce). However, there is a solution to this problem in the form of monounsaturated fats. These fats, as mentioned previously, are derived from olive oil and avocado oil. Monounsaturated fats have the capacity to reduce the level of LDL but allow the beneficial HDL to remain the same.

This may explain why the so-called Mediterranean diet has such a good reputation for its health-enhancing properties and in particular, for protecting the heart, since this diet is rich in olive oil in addition to garlic. Sports people will also be interested to know that exercise has been shown to improve HDL levels.

Hydrogenated fat

As a result of the cholesterol scare, millions of people switched from butter to margarine. However, it is worth noting that a lot of margarine products on the market contain hydrogenated fat. Such fat is produced by the manufacturer when hydrogen is introduced into the polyunsaturated fats, this converts them into solid fats. As mentioned previously in this book, consumption of such margarine or other products containing hydrogenated fats (e.g. some biscuits) may encourage the production of free radicals which are associated with cell destruction in the body. Fortunately an increasing number of manufacturers are switching to non-hydrogenated fats, so you may wish to check this out by carefully scrutinising food labels.

Getting the balance of fats right

As the reader will have observed from the foregoing information on saturated and polyunsaturated fats, it is not only important to eat less saturated fat in favour of the polyunsaturated type. It is also important to include monounsaturated fats in the diet. Many nutritionists are now advocating one-third saturated fat, one-third polyunsaturated fat and one-third monounsaturated fat.

There are a number of oil mixes currently on the market which are derived from vegetable oils. These can be taken as a supplement. They should always be cold pressed and kept in an airtight container in the fridge. When taking such oils, I would personally recommend that you increase your level of vitamin E, which will help to complement their effect.

Some key points about fat consumption

There is no necessity to entirely eliminate saturated fats from the diet. However, they should be kept to a minimum, with greater emphasis being placed upon polyunsaturated fats and monounsaturated fats. Monounsaturated fats from olive oil and avocados are particularly beneficial to the heart and circulatory system and should be incorporated into the everyday diet.

Avoid the folly of adhering to a virtually fat-free diet in order to lose weight. People who do this risk a deterioration in their health because fats have important functions in the body. So remember, low fat not no fat!

Do try to incorporate olive oil into your diet. It can be used in cooking or added to salads (for example, in a home made French dressing). The best olive oil is extra virgin, preferably cold pressed in order to preserve its nutritional value.

Both fats and oils have the same calorific value. This should be taken into account when working out energy values.

If you are a vegetarian it may be worth considering the inclusion of flax seed oil, or a supplement of cold pressed oils (preferably from organic sources) which will provide a broad spectrum of EFAs, including the omega 3 fatty acids.

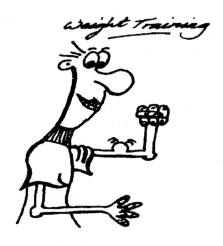

CHAPTER 14   WEIGHT TRAINING: ITS ROLE IN THE NATURAL ATHLETE'S LIFESTYLE

Weight training can play a pivotal role in the overall lifestyle of sportsmen and women. As a means of enhancing physical performance and even helping to prevent some injuries, I would rate weight training as second in importance only to nutrition.

Now in my forties, I attempt to train four or five times each week. I spend approximately forty five minutes in the gym during each session and not hours on end like some people. However, my time in the gym is quality time and my programme is short but intensive. This produces good results and helps me avoid over-training - a common mistake these days, since many mistakenly equate quantity of training with quality. The beauty of weight training is that it can help you to look good and feel good way into old age.

When in my twenties I was inspired by an Australian athlete called Percy Cerutty. In his seventies, he not only ran many miles each week, but trained religiously with weights, exhibiting feats of strength and endurance which would have shamed many men half his age. His excellent book: 'Be fit or Be Damned', in my opinion, was way ahead of its time. Undoubtedly, Percy Cerutty was an enlightened man; very well educated on the subject of nutrition, he epitomised the lifestyle of the natural athlete. Way before the idea of eating the correct foods in the right balance in order to prolong an active life and maximise performance was widely accepted, Percy Cerruty was a shining example to sports people everywhere. He was also aware of the preventative role that diet plays in helping us to build a greater resistance to chronic diseases such as cancer, diabetes and heart disease.

Even today, some people think of weight training as an activity for the younger person. Studies in countries such as America have proven such beliefs to be erroneous. Studies of resistance training programmes for the elderly have shown amazing results with people between the ages of seventy and ninety-eight, showing significant improvements in strength, stamina and general muscle tone. Other similar studies have shown that weight training improves metabolism, sleep quality, digestion and bone density.

In light of this information, I am reminded of the old adage 'use it or lose it'. Remember, the body has evolved over millions of years as a machine that needs hard work. It has been designed to thrive on activity, without it the body will deteriorate. Without regular suitable activity it has been shown that the body will lose approximately five to seven pounds of lean tissue every ten years. This process can be largely averted if we engage in regular weight training. Another benefit of weight training is that it helps us to remain in good shape. This in itself gives us a beneficial psychological boost, since if we look good we feel good, and in later years, you will feel a sense of achievement at having reversed the ageing process.

Training for best results

Sadly most people in gyms don't train correctly. Firstly, they will avoid hard work wherever possible. Let's face it, we all seek the 'least line of resistance' whenever possible. However, the fact is that no real improvement will ensue in terms of muscle mass and/or muscle tone, unless a degree of discomfort is experienced. Therefore, the adage 'no pain, no gain' is true, although this is obviously relevant to the age and personal objectives of the individual. I always work on the principle that your last repetition on a given exercise should be a struggle so that another repetition is not possible. Only when this point is reached will muscle strength increase.

When performing an exercise it is best to do it in good style, that is to say, without cheating movements when other muscles try to help out. This only defeats the object of the exercise, which is to provide quality resistance to the muscle being exercised. Only then will maximum results ensue.

Many gym enthusiasts cheat by doing each repetition too quickly. It's always easier to perform quick repetitions instead of slower ones. Try comparing a slow press-up to a fast one and you'll soon see the difference. The ideal time it takes to complete a repetition is five seconds - two seconds out, a brief pause and two to three seconds to return the weight to its original starting position. This ensures that the muscle is worked properly over its full range of movement. Weight trainers who find that it is easier to do small movements which allow them to shift more weight are just kidding themselves. Far better to use less weight and do the exercise correctly. This will result in gradual but steady improvement.

If you are seeking to reduce your waistline, then do not expect endless sit-ups to do the job. Yes, the abdominal muscles will be stronger and this in itself is desirable, but to lose inches from the waist, combine exercise with a reduced calorie intake. Sensible eating and proper exercise, as already discussed, are major factors in the lifestyle of the natural athlete. Those wishing to gain strength should aim to eat several small meals a day instead of three large ones. This is because the body can only ingest a certain amount of protein from each meal, and since protein is essential for building muscle this is an important consideration when planning your daily dietary programme. Remember though, the pitfalls involved in consuming too much protein, as discussed earlier in this book.

Injury prevention
Perhaps it sounds a little absurd to think in terms of helping to prevent injury. Let's face it, some injuries are not preventable. When we think of that horrendous injury sustained by Paul Gascoigne in the FA Cup Final it's hard to think of him coming out of such a suicidal tackle unscathed. Perhaps the only thing that could have saved Gascoigne from all the pain, frustration and months of gruelling physiotherapy that ensued from that moment of reckless abandon, would have been self-restraint. Nevertheless, leaving this kind of incident aside, I believe that weight training does have a role to play in injury prevention. Perhaps this assertion is best illustrated by a story I came across when I was in my late teens. It concerned a young man, possibly in his mid-twenties, who had worked hard with weights in order to build up a powerful physique. Being involved in the sport of wrestling he had spent some time in order to develop his neck muscles, a practice not uncommon with wrestlers. Unfortunately, one day he was involved in a serious car crash and as a result sustained some serious injuries. What was particularly interesting, however, is that the consultant who was dealing with the case stated that if it had not been for this man's powerful physique and unusually strong neck, he would, in his opinion, have surely been killed.

In essence, we can conclude from this story that if muscles, tendons and ligaments which surround the joints of the body are strengthened, then a greater chance of protection will be afforded by those joints in the event of physical trauma occurring. An example of this would be a rugby player being tackled sideways-on, and a lot of stress being placed on the knee joint. What tends to happen in such cases is a tightening of the muscles surrounding the joint, resulting in greater stability. If these muscles are well developed, as a result of progressive weight training, then the joint is capable of tolerating greater stress. This will either result in no injury occurring or a significantly less severe injury taking place. This is obviously of immense benefit to the individual concerned.

Weight training, therefore, does have a place in the overall training programme, both in terms of helping to prevent or minimise injury and also in order to enhance physical performance. Furthermore, its versatility cannot be underestimated, since, even when an injury takes place, an athlete can still continue to train in a controlled manner in order to aid recovery. For example, in the past, whenever I have sustained a leg injury, usually as a result of playing football, I have continued to do upper body training. Also, when movement is possible in the injured limb (i.e. when it is relatively pain free) then training can be geared towards aiding a quicker recovery.

The importance of quality stretching
Having underlined the benefits of progressive weight training, it is important to remember that regardless of your chosen sport, it is essential that you take a few minutes each day in order to do stretching exercises. The importance of stretching should be stressed to all sports participants, including children and adults of all ages. If children are taught the value of stretching early on, they will benefit in the sense of building up an increased resistance to injury and also greater flexibility when adulthood is reached.

The aim of stretching is to increase and maintain flexibility of the tendons and ligaments which surround the joints of the body. Bearing in mind the aforementioned information about strengthening support structures that surround joints, it is important to remember that the stability of these bodily structures will be further enhanced if a good degree of flexibility is also introduced. This stands to reason, since if a joint is both strong and flexible at the same time, then when stress is placed upon the joint (e.g. the shoulder joint in a javelin thrower) the end result is a greater capacity to resist injury. Moreover, the greater range of movement that will ensue as a result of the improved flexibility will help to improve performance. Again, the javelin thrower serves as a good example, because a greater range of movement results in the force behind the throw being exerted over a greater range. Hence the strength of the throw should increase. This is one reason why we observe sprinters spending so much time before a race warming up and stretching, since flexibility of the hips and legs is so important. Also, and equally important, we need to ensure that tendons, muscles and ligaments are warmed up and pliable since we are very prone to injury when these structures are placed under sudden stress when cold. To visualise this, just imagine an elastic band which has been placed in a fridge for a few hours. When stretched it will be much more likely to snap. The same elastic band when left in a warm environment will have a greater capacity to stretch before snapping.

Being involved in different sports on a day to day basis, I often observe people making basic mistakes when stretching. The most common error is that of stretching before warming up - remember the elastic band analogy. The pattern for pre-activity stretching should be as follows:

1. Aerobic activity, e.g. gentle jogging, skipping etc.
2. Stretching all major joints commencing with the ankles and working upwards through the knees, hips, spine, shoulders etc.
3. More vigorous aerobic activity, e.g. 3/4 pace running, long stride running, moving side to side etc.
4. Further stretching, holding for approximately 15 to 20 seconds on each stretch.

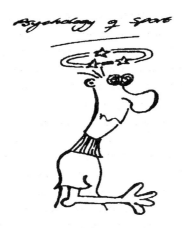

CHAPTER 15   SPORTS PSYCHOLOGY

Visualise, if you will, two opposing tennis players who, in terms of ability and athleticism, are identical. The only difference between them is that one player has a mental edge. He not only has more self-belief, he has a greater will to win. There would be no prizes for guessing which player is likely to be victorious.

The role that the mind plays in terms of sporting success is now recognised more than ever before. In the last Olympic games the athletes representing their respective countries were accompanied by a number of sports psychologists. The objective was to help the athletes mentally prepare for the competition ahead. This preparation includes a number of mind techniques which can be employed by the athlete, not only before an event, but also during competition itself.

I have recently been very privileged to become acquainted with the hypnotherapist Glenn Harrold. He frequently works with children and adults; helping them to develop a positive approach towards their chosen sport. He uses hypnotherapy in order to aid the mind in accepting positive suggestions, designed to improve performance. As Glenn pointed out to me, the mind is similar to a computer, if you 'feed it' with certain information, this is then stored in the subconscious memory, to be recalled whenever required. By exposing the mind to a number of appropriate positive suggestions, positive thought is transferred into positive action; for example, in relation to football, the suggestions might be'I will accelerate past an opposing player, I will always remain composed under pressure, I will be positive and confident at all times'.

By placing emphasis upon only positive aspects of a particular sport and taking steps to eradicate any negative thoughts, such as 'maybe I won't score from this penalty', then overall performance will often improve.

Of course, it would be true to say that some sportsmen and women already possess an inherent self-belief and positive attitude when engaged in competitive sport. One has only to look at the attitude exhibited by Mohammed Ali, who some would argue, was the world's greatest ever boxer. He often had an edge over opponents before a punch was even exchanged. This was due to his ability to portray an image of sheer invincibility. Linford Christie, one of the world's greatest sprinters, also possessed great self-belief; and furthermore, like many world class athletes, Linford had the ability to cut out all peripheral distractions and remain entirely focused upon the task ahead.

This ability to focus and exclude noise and other potential distractions is very evident when we observe people such as the world class tennis player Steffi Graf. Some tennis players have a habit of dwelling upon a close line call, or a missed opportunity when attempting to win the point. Steffi Graf, however, was more apt to forget the last point and focus on the point ahead. Such an approach helps to ensure that a player doesn't 'beat himself up' by dwelling upon what cannot be changed.

Mental imagery
Glenn Harrold taught me that mental imagery is a useful tool when it comes to winning in sport. For instance, whilst taking one of my regular coaching sessions with the junior team that I manage, I made a point of

addressing the importance of adopting the correct mental attitude when attempting to score goals. I asked the players to imagine that every time they got an opportunity to shoot at goal they could visualise themselves scoring the perfect goal every time. I explained to the players that of course they wouldn't always score. However, I also helped them to understand that by using such imagery in conjunction with adopting a positive attitude, the percentage of goals scored in relation to attempts on goal would significantly increase. I further explained that footballers such as Michael Owen and Alan Shearer may also use such visualisation techniques in order to help them achieve a greater success rate. Furthermore, this same principle can be applied to all aspects of sporting endeavour; for example, the high jumper making the perfect jump or the javelin thrower achieving a personal best.

Such mental imaging in conjunction with auto-suggestion represent powerful tools in terms of achieving an improving level of success in sport.

The following 'star performer profile' helps to illustrate this point, and as can be observed, the mental aspect of an individual's sporting development is very significant.

Star Performer - A Profile:

1. Physique:
    a) good agility
    b) all round strength
    c) mobility

2. Fitness:
    a) cardiovascular
    b) endurance/stamina
    c) recovery

3. Technique:
   a) technical ability
   b) ability to conceptualise motor movements
   c) ability to put into effect in training/matches

4. Vision - reading the game:
   a) tactical ability
   b) visualising one or more moves ahead

5. Mental:
   a) self-belief
   b) ability to focus attention (e.g. in tennis, on the next point)
   c) ability to blank out external distractions
   d) ability to use visionary and other self-hypnotic techniques
   e) will to win
   f) hunger for success
   g) ability to remain in control (keep your cool) under pressure
   h) ability to accept defeat as a learning experience and platform
      for future improvement

6. Work rate:
   a) ability to maintain high work rate in training and matches

7. Fulfilment:
   a) enjoyment/love of the game

When we look at the athlete as a composite being, composed of both physical and mental aspects, it becomes clear why a holistic approach towards training and performance is so important. Of course, depending upon your personal beliefs, some would add a spiritual component to the equation, perceiving the athlete as a combination of physical, mental and spiritual aspects. Certainly, some athletes feel that their own religious beliefs have provided them with greater inner strength, which in turn has helped them to achieve more success in their chosen sport. When Cassius Clay changed his religion and his name to Mohammed Ali, his personal religious conviction undoubtedly provided him with immense inner strength and conviction when encountering highly respected world class boxing opponents.

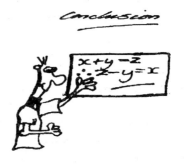

CHAPTER 16   CONCLUSION

If the foregoing information concerning the importance of diet in relation to health promotion and enhancement of athletic performance is to be given any credence, it could perhaps be argued that certain conclusions need to drawn and subsequently acted upon.

Despite the dietary differences that exist from one person to the next, for example, food intolerance towards a specific food, there would appear to be certain common dietary principles that apply to the vast majority of people. If we pay a visit to a doctor's surgery, hospital or clinic, we are often the recipient of a multitude of health messages, many of which relate to diet and health. Not too long ago the connection was thought to be far too tenuous to be broadcast in the form of posters, information leaflets and so on. The concept of 'we are what we eat' would seem to have been merely a 'crankish' idea confined to a minority of health conscious people.

In the light of current scientific evidence, it would appear that the public perception of what constitutes a healthy diet may be slowly changing. Publications such as the World Health Organisation Report on 'Diet, Nutrition and the Prevention of Chronic Diseases' may continue to sway public opinion in favour of healthy eating. Consistent with the recommendations of the aforementioned NACNE and COMA reports, according to this article which appeared in the 'Health Guardian', the report states the following:

> "A major recommendation is the advice that everyone should consume 400g (almost one pound) of fresh fruit and vegetables every day - this is to include pulses, nuts and seeds, but to exclude potatoes and other tuber vegetables. This recommendation is based on observed intakes of fruit and vegetables in regions such as Southern Italy or parts of Greece, where high intakes are associated with low rates of chronic diseases and also on medical studies into nutrient deficiencies"

Health Guardian, Fresh Advice on Fruit, 1991, page 1.

If we relate these latest recommendations to the findings from previous research, it is interesting to note that the similarities are marked.

Even as far back as the 1930s, pioneers such as Sir Robert McCarrison were conducting research projects which added to the accumulating evidence that the western diet was inextricably linked with the causation of diseases such as certain cancers, heart disease, high blood pressure and diabetes.

To many present day sports people unacquainted with the importance of good dietary principles, these are perhaps remote concepts extremely far removed from training schedules, competitions and matches. It is my express hope, therefore, that this book may help to fill a gap, albeit a small one, in order that all those involved in the business of sport, may at least be stimulated to think about their general lifestyle and diet. It is also to be hoped that such introspection and subsequent assessment of the subject of diet and sports performance may prompt the reader of this book to make positive changes in order to not only enhance their chances of attaining optimum performance, but also to maintain general health and well-being throughout life.

Perhaps it is a fitting conclusion to this work that I end here with a poem which I wrote called 'Heritage of Health'. In many ways it embodies much of what this book is all about.

HERITAGE OF HEALTH

Chemicals on your crops, pollution in the air,
Junk food on the menu, no-one seems to care,
Nitrates in your water, plutonium on the land,
Fast food in your trolley, Choose your favourite brand.
Sewage in your oceans, acid in the lake,
Mercury in your tuna, so many lives at stake.

Cholesterol for dinner, cholesterol for tea,
Cholesterol for supper, no friend of artery.
Sugar on my cornflakes, sugar for my tea,
Sugar makes the journey sweet, to the cemetery.
Junk food for ever, yes sir if you please,
Steel yourself for cancer, and a dose of heart disease.

But as I look around me, at a world gone mad,
I know to cherish nature is no passing fad.
So dream the dream of sanity, restored to all around,
When crops grow as times gone by, in unpolluted ground.
And Mother Nature, now reborn, the air like still of night,
Our heritage of health renewed, no more this earthly blight.

APPENDIX

The following dietary suggestions were constructed in order to help Jamie Johnson make the transition from a diet which consisted mainly of refined foods, to one which comprised of wholefoods. Consideration has also been given to the acid/alkaline balance. The principal aim was to help her body to eliminate toxins, restore the acid/alkaline balance, boost her immune system and provide enough protein and carbohydrate to supply her energy requirements for professional boxing:

HEALTHY FOOD IDEAS

Muesli

This is good if eaten with at least equal quantities of fruit. I suggest you soak the muesli in semi-skimmed organic milk (goat's or cow's); or try goat's yoghurt sweetened with a little honey or dried fruit.

Tuna Sandwich

Best made with 100% wholewheat bread (preferably organic). Balance this with either fruit or salad.

NB. You might wish to experiment with different healthy sandwich fillings, such as vegetarian paté with alfalfa sprouts (which are rich in protein and nutrients).

Soup

This can be good for your new healthy lifestyle, but select only natural soups (packet soups are usually out, since they contain too many chemicals!). I strongly recommend organic soups. When buying them, look at the ingredients; a lot of manufacturers include sugar and white flour, so try to avoid these. Alternatively, you can make a batch of soup at home and take this to the gym in a thermos flask. It makes a nourishing lunch, eaten with wholewheat or rye.

Fish and Rice

Use wholegrain rice (the brown variety) and add fish, such as cod or tuna. Deep-sea fish are usually safer to eat, since most fish caught close to coastlines are likely to be more polluted.

Toast and Marmite
This is good when using wholewheat bread. Marmite is a good source of B vitamins and vegetable protein.

Jacket Potato
Choose organic potatoes if possible (you wouldn't believe what they spray ordinary potatoes with!). Good fillings include cottage cheese, baked beans and tuna. Balance with salad or vegetables.

HEALTHY MEAL IDEAS
BREAKFAST
Fruit, muesli with organic semi-skimmed milk or organic soya milk.

OR: Marmite on toast and fresh fruit.

OR: Porridge made with organic oats and milk, sweetened with a little honey or dried fruit (e.g. organic dates or raisins).

OR: soaked organic dried fruit, such as raisins, sultanas, dates and apricots (you can leave these to soak the night before and eat them in the morning). Have with some organic soya milk or yoghurt.

LUNCH
Organic soup with wholemeal bread, spread with a little butter or cold-pressed margarine. Follow with some fresh fruit.

OR: Tuna sandwich made with wholemeal or rye bread. Balance with fruit or salad.

OR: Mixed salad – this can be prepared the night before in a plastic sealed container. Keep it in the fridge overnight and take to the gym the next day.

Examples Of Ingredients: grated carrots, celery, apple, beetroot, raisins, onions, sunflower seeds, chopped ice-burg lettuce, bean sprouts (such as alfalfa), nuts, tuna, brown rice, etc.

Dressing: you can make your own using cider vinegar and olive oil. The composition is one part vinegar to two parts oil. Or buy a ready-made dressing; there are lots of healthy brands to choose from.

EVENING MEAL

Brown rice, tuna, onions, plenty of vegetables.

Dessert: fruit, or an organic soya dessert.

OR: Large stir-fry. You can include lots of different vegetables (preferably organic, either frozen or fresh). Add to this some chicken or fish for protein. Flavour with organic stock or soya sauce.

Dessert: organic ice-cream or soya dessert.

OR: Wholemeal pasta flavoured with organic pasta sauce. Add a little grated cow's or goat's cheese. Eat with a salad or your favourite vegetables.

OR: jacket potato with cottage cheese, beans and a salad.

Dessert: fruit.

OR: Large mixed salad made up in a salad bowl. Be adventurous and experiment with ingredients. Add some wholemeal pasta and chunks of organic cheese, and have with a natural dressing.

HEALTHY SNACKS

Choosing healthy snacks will give you energy between meals, but only eat when feeling hungry. Try nibbling on some pumpkin or sunflower seeds, a piece of fruit, or carrot sticks, etc.

WATER

Try to avoid tap water – it contains too many chemicals! Choose instead spring, mineral or filtered water. Drinking lots of pure water will help to eliminate toxins and hydrate your system, which will help your boxing performance.

DETOX SYMPTOMS

Remember not to worry about any of the detox symptoms we've already discussed. These are a good sign and mean your body is getting rid of toxins (poisons), which have the potential of affecting your health and training. Once your system has cleared itself of these toxins, you will feel a lot healthier and have a greater resistance to illness. This will be reflected in your physical stamina and general fitness.

SPECIAL NOTE

The aforementioned dietary suggestions were made for Jamie following her visit to Signs Of Life, where she was tested for any food intolerances which may have been present. This meant that foods such as soya and a variety of grains, could be included in her diet. If you know of any food intolerances or allergies (for example to peanuts), which affect you, then I suggest you adhere to a similar diet as outlined in the foregoing, whilst remembering to make suitable substitutions for any problem foods.

Recommended Reading

Magazines

The Vitamin Connection   International Magazine of Health and
Fitness, Alphavite Publications Ltd.
Health and Fitness   Finsbury Business Centre.
Here's Health   Greater London House, Hampstead Road,
London, NW1 7EJ

Books

McCarrison, R, and Sinclair, H.M. 1936, Nutrition and Health, Faber
and Faber.
Walker, N.W., 1976, Raw Vegetable Juices, Pyramid Books, New York.
Burkitt, D., 1979, Don't Forget Fibre In Your Diet, Martin Dunit Ltd.
Baker, G.H.,1975, Keep Healthy Stay Younger.
Vogel, A., 1977, The Nature Doctor, Verlag. Vogel, Switzerland.
Kenton, L., 1989 Ageless Ageing, Century Arrow.
Holford, P., 1997, The Optimum Nutrition Bible, Piatkus

Government Publications

Great Britain, DHSS,1964,The COMA Report, HMSO, London.
Health Education Council,1963, The NACNE Report.

Useful Addresses

Glenn Harrold - Diviniti Publishing - Glenn Harrold - Hypnotherapist.
Diviniti Publishing Ltd., 6 Elm Walk, Aylesford, Kent, ME20 7LS.

Index